Athletic Fitness for Kids

Scott Lancaster

Radu Teodorescu

Human Kinetics

Library of Congress Cataloging-in-Publication Data

Lancaster, Scott B.
  Athletic fitness for kids / Scott Lancaster, Radu Teodorescu.
    p. cm.
  ISBN-13: 978-0-7360-6242-8 (soft cover)
  ISBN-10: 0-7360-6242-4 (soft cover)
  1. Physical fitness for children. 2. Physical education for children.
  I. Teodorescu, Radu, 1944- II. Title.
  GV443.L32 2008
  613.7'042--dc22

                              2007026598

ISBN-10: 0-7360-6242-4
ISBN-13: 978-0-7360-6242-8

This publication is written and published to provide accurate and authoritative information relevant to the subject matter presented. It is published and sold with the understanding that the author and publisher are not engaged in rendering legal, medical, or other professional services by reason of their authorship or publication of this work. If medical or other expert assistance is required, the services of a competent professional person should be sought.

The Web addresses cited in this text were current as of July, 2007, unless otherwise noted.

Acquisitions Editor: Laurel Plotzke; **Developmental Editor:** Amanda Eastin-Allen; **Assistant Editor:** Christine Horger; **Copyeditor:** John Wentworth; **Proofreader:** Jim Burns; **Graphic Designer:** Fred Starbird; **Graphic Artist:** Tara Welsch; **Cover Designer:** Keith Blomberg; **Photographer (cover):** Neil Bernstein; **Photographer (interior):** Dennis Fagan unless otherwise noted; photos on pp. 3, 11, 18, 40, 64, 82, 102, 122 and 144 © Human Kinetics; **Photo Asset Manager:** Laura Fitch; **Art Manager:** Kelly Hendren; **Associate Art Manager:** Alan L. Wilborn; **Illustrator:** Accurate Art; **Printer:** United Graphics

Human Kinetics books are available at special discounts for bulk purchase. Special editions or book excerpts can also be created to specification. For details, contact the Special Sales Manager at Human Kinetics.

Printed in the United States of America   10 9 8 7 6 5

The paper in this book is certified under a sustainable forestry program.

Human Kinetics
Web site: www.HumanKinetics.com

United States: Human Kinetics
P.O. Box 5076
Champaign, IL 61825-5076
800-747-4457
e-mail: humank@hkusa.com

Canada: Human Kinetics
475 Devonshire Road, Unit 100
Windsor, ON N8Y 2L5
800-465-7301 (in Canada only)
e-mail: info@hkcanada.com

Europe: Human Kinetics
107 Bradford Road
Stanningley
Leeds LS28 6AT, United Kingdom
+44 (0)113 255 5665
e-mail: hk@hkeurope.com

Australia: Human Kinetics
57A Price Avenue
Lower Mitcham, South Australia 5062
08 8372 0999
e-mail: info@hkaustralia.com

New Zealand: Human Kinetics
P.O. Box 80
Torrens Park, South Australia 5062
0800 222 062
e-mail: info@hknewzealand.com

Athletic Fitness
for Kids

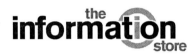

the
information
store

**Please return on or before
the last date stamped below.
Contact:** 01603 773 114
or 01603 773 224

2 5 IAN 2017

243 793

This book is for my son, Justin, whose passion for play always inspires me to want to do more for him and his generation. And for my wife, Susan, whose love, support, and understanding made this journey a success.

—Scott Lancaster

I dedicate this book to Alexander and Andrew, my sons, for their support and inspiration. The experience I had with them during the hungry athletic years made it easier to write this book and convinced me of the realistic need for such a book in every family.

—Radu Teodorescu

Contents

Drill Finder

Drill #	Drill	Sport application							Page #
		Baseball	Basketball	Football	Hockey	Lacrosse	Soccer	Tennis	
Flexibility									
3.1	Obstacle Course Warm-Up	✔		✔		✔	✔		23
3.2	Front Shoulder ROM	✔	✔	✔	✔	✔	✔	✔	24
3.3	Top of Shoulder ROM	✔	✔	✔	✔	✔	✔	✔	25
3.4	Posterior Shoulder ROM	✔	✔	✔	✔	✔	✔	✔	26
3.5	Side of Hip ROM	✔	✔	✔	✔	✔	✔	✔	27
3.6	Front and Side of Hip ROM	✔	✔	✔	✔	✔	✔	✔	28
3.7	Static Stretches	✔	✔	✔	✔	✔	✔	✔	30
3.8	Soccer Warm-Up						✔		35
3.9	Tennis Warm-Up							✔	36
Coordination									
4.1	Stomp and Clap	✔	✔	✔	✔	✔	✔	✔	42
4.2	Reactive Knee Lifts	✔	✔	✔	✔	✔	✔	✔	43
4.3	Multidirectional Lunges	✔	✔	✔	✔	✔	✔	✔	45
4.4	Coordinated Skips	✔	✔	✔	✔	✔	✔	✔	46
4.5	Eye–Foot Coordination			✔	✔		✔	✔	47
4.6	Circle Dribbling				✔		✔	✔	50
4.7	Lower-Body Juggling			✔	✔	✔	✔	✔	51
4.8	Spot the Ball	✔			✔	✔		✔	53
4.9	In Motion Hand–Eye Coordination	✔	✔	✔	✔	✔		✔	56
4.10	Football Coordination			✔					58
4.11	Lacrosse Coordination					✔			60

Drill #	Drill	Sport application							Page #
		Baseball	Basketball	Football	Hockey	Lacrosse	Soccer	Tennis	
Balance									
5.1	Balance in Motion	✔	✔	✔	✔	✔	✔	✔	65
5.2	Knee Balancing	✔	✔	✔	✔	✔	✔	✔	68
5.3	Balance Boarding	✔	✔	✔	✔	✔	✔	✔	70
5.4	Balancing in Different Body Positions	✔	✔	✔	✔	✔	✔	✔	71
5.5	Bicycle Balance	✔	✔	✔	✔	✔	✔	✔	72
5.6	Roll, Balance, and Run			✔	✔	✔	✔		76
5.7	Tennis Balancing							✔	78
5.8	Basketball Balancing		✔	✔	✔				79
Stamina									
6.1	Stamina Course for Younger Kids	✔	✔	✔	✔	✔	✔	✔	84
6.2	Stamina Course for Older Kids	✔	✔	✔	✔	✔	✔	✔	86
6.3	Track Run	✔	✔	✔	✔	✔	✔	✔	88
6.4	Up and Down Track	✔	✔	✔	✔	✔	✔	✔	89
6.5	On- and Off-Track	✔	✔	✔	✔	✔	✔	✔	90
6.6	Water Running	✔	✔	✔	✔	✔	✔	✔	93
6.7	Ultimate Frisbee	✔	✔	✔	✔	✔	✔	✔	93
6.8	Baseball Stamina	✔							94
6.9	Football Stamina	✔							97

Drill #	Drill	Sport application							Page #
		Baseball	Basketball	Football	Hockey	Lacrosse	Soccer	Tennis	
		Agility							
9.1	Body Awareness and Control	✔	✔	✔	✔	✔	✔	✔	145
9.2	Three-Legged Moves	✔	✔	✔	✔	✔	✔	✔	147
9.3	Multiple and Continuous Movements	✔	✔	✔	✔	✔	✔	✔	148
9.4	Quick Feet	✔	✔	✔	✔	✔	✔	✔	151
9.5	Crossing the Feet	✔	✔	✔	✔	✔	✔	✔	154
9.6	30-Yard Athletic Slalom			✔		✔	✔		156
9.7	Stop, Cut, and Go			✔		✔	✔		158
9.8	Run & Shoot and Run & Throw	✔		✔		✔	✔		159
9.9	Soccer Agility		✔		✔		✔	✔	160

Acknowledgments

I would like to thank my editors, Laurel Plotzke and Mandy Eastin-Allen, for their patience and dedication to the entire project. I also am very grateful to Martin Barnard for believing in this project and signing me on to Human Kinetics.

As with any book, there is always a need to have a strong team of people that gets things done. Lee Becker was one such person who was always there in the clutch to make things happen. Thanks to the town of Basking Ridge, New Jersey, for so graciously hosting our photo shoot. I am also grateful to all the kids that spent a very warm day patiently demonstrating all the drills for our photographer. Thank you to my hometown of Somers, New York, and Roman Catalino for hosting my many clinics that helped develop and shape the premise of this book.

A special thanks to all the people at CapRio Management for their support and for believing in the overall vision of this project.

Thanks to Steve Cohen, vice president of Sirius Radio Sports Programming, as well as Sirius NFL hosts Tim Ryan and Pat Kirwan for giving me the forum to extend my youth sports solutions to so many parents and coaches nationwide on the *ABCs of Sports* and the Sirius NFL program, *Movin' the Chains*.

Also, thanks to Bill Maier and Sean Brawley for their support and insight throughout the entire writing process.

Finally, thanks to Mike Wiocik for his unique and creative approach to the teaching and coaching that he extended to me as my track coach at Syracuse University. Mike's innovative approach awakened me to the many different and creative ways athletes can learn and improve performance.

—Scott Lancaster

I would like to thank the editors, Laurel Plotzke and Mandy Eastin-Allen, for their dedication, patience, and support during the entire project.

—Radu Teodorescu

CHAPTER 1

The Athletic Fitness Method

All sports are based on athletes moving in the most effective ways they can to perform skills that apply to their sport. For athletes to improve and excel in a sport, they need to experience how their bodies should react while executing sport-specific moves. If they don't get this experience, they have a distinct disadvantage when the time comes to take the field or court. For example, a young baseball player might be trained in the basics of fielding a ground ball but not know how to efficiently move to the ball from various directions. This book is designed to prepare young athletes for athletic situations so that they can execute sport-specific techniques with confidence and ease. It's our hope that our methods of instruction will keep more young athletes participating in their sport of choice and that they will continue to grow in confidence and ability as they mature.

Our athletic fitness method focuses on essential movement fundamentals *for the entire body* to best prepare young athletes for sport participation. In this chapter we'll discuss what our athletic component program consists of, how our method improves sport-specific skills, and the benefits of integrating our program into your young athletes' athletic training.

WHAT IS AN ATHLETIC FITNESS PROGRAM?

An athletic fitness program is a fun, creative approach to improving athletic abilities. Our program breaks fundamentals down into seven athletic components essential for success in any sport. These components are flexibility, coordination, balance, stamina, strength, speed, and agility. Our program helps athletes improve in each of these seven areas, the result being a much more well-rounded and physically and mentally prepared athlete.

By incorporating movement training from all areas of fitness into your practices or training sessions, you enable your athletes to develop overall athletic movements that will help improve on the basic execution of sport-specific techniques, and thus improve on overall performance. Collectively, the proper introduction and development of these athletic components give young athletes the foundation to achieve their potential in any sport they choose. With efficacy in the seven athletic components, athletes will find themselves able to execute important game-specific fundamentals such as throwing on the run (agility, balance, coordination); avoiding multiple defenders (agility, speed, coordination); bunting a baseball (coordination); maintaining possession after taking a hit in soccer, hockey, or lacrosse (agility, balance); battling for a puck in hockey (strength, coordination); or chasing a pass down the wing at the end of a soccer game (stamina, speed), to name just a few.

A core theory behind an athletic fitness program, and behind this book, is the necessary elimination of traditional, noncontemporary methods of training. The goal of our method is to help you creatively present and structure training in ways that young athletes find enjoyable and entertaining. In our program, training is implemented through fun drills and activities that provide opportunities for self-testing and self-measurement of progress and success. Unique to our approach is that everyone can participate and challenge themselves in a nonstressful way. Athletes repeatedly practice to improve, measuring themselves against set standards and their own past performances. This is an approach commonly seen in sports such as skateboarding, boogie-boarding, surfing, and trick cycling in which athletes strive to improve on their own standards of success. Through our approach, athletes benefit by enjoying experiential learning through progressive challenges that are not critically judged by others. Rather, athletes assess themselves through a process of self-awareness and correction within a fun, yet competitive, environment.

In this book, each of the seven fundamental athletic components is devoted its own chapter that includes drills and self-competitions to allow athletes to track and measure their progress. The drills use English measurements. For metric equivalents, refer to Appendix A in the back of the book. The chapters describe the proper technique to execute each skill, how to incorporate athletic equipment and adjust to an environment, and ways of introducing a combination of variables that help athletes adapt to athletic situations they'll face when executing the skill in competition. For example, we discuss how to develop speed not only for linear pursuits but for situations that call for athletes to move in multiple directions, suddenly stopping, and then restarting. We recommend introducing your athletes to several exercises from each chapter at a time and using the self-competitions to measure their progress.

What you won't find in this book is specific skill instruction by sport. To enhance the development of your young athletes' sport-specific skills, we recommend incorporating our athletic fitness training methods

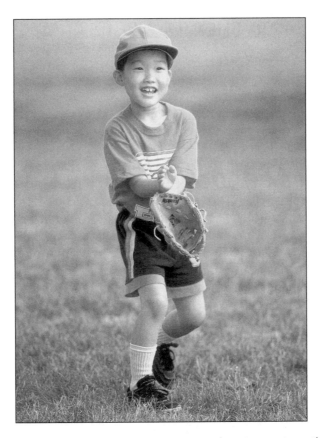

An athletic fitness program is a fun, creative approach to improving athletic abilities by incorporating movement training from all areas of fitness.

before and throughout sport-specific training. Athletes who feel comfortable with their abilities on the field or court will have a consistent and clear advantage throughout their athletic careers. If athletes struggle with increasing their speed, developing agility, maintaining strength, keeping balance, or building stamina, no amount of sport-specific training will significantly improve their athletic performance. The continued development of general movement skills is a major part of professional training, both in season and off season.

Instead of sport-specific instruction, what this book delivers is a variety of drills and activities that replicate sport-specific skill movements found in baseball, basketball, football, hockey, lacrosse, soccer, and tennis. These sport-specific drills directly apply to the athletic components we feature and are provided to give you an idea of how to apply the athletic component to an athlete's particular sport in a practice or training session. Appendix B does provide some sport-specific throwing tips to help young athletes properly execute the throwing skills employed in the drills and competitions found in this book.

WHY YOU SHOULD USE OUR METHOD

By integrating our method into your training of your young athletes (or your own children), you will see improved creativity and individuality in their athletic skills and all related sport-specific skills. You'll also witness significant improvements in their overall fitness levels.

Next time you attend a youth athletic event, focus on how the children move. Watch how they run up and down the court or field and how they jump, kick, and throw. You will see that some kids excel while others look awkward and out of place. This is because some children are well trained in fundamental movement, and others lack even the most basic athletic skills. Even at the high school varsity level you might see baseball players and quarterbacks with poor throwing mechanics, basketball players who don't jump correctly, football players who can't get themselves into a proper stance, or track athletes with poor running form. The fact is that many athletes don't reach their true natural athletic potential and never achieve their ultimate peak performance because they didn't learn the basics when they were young.

Gone are the days when nearly every child experienced physical activity on every day they attended school. Today, students are lucky to get an hour of any type of organized physical activity in a week. Kids today are living in a technologically advanced society that promotes sedentary habits and has diminished appreciation for physical activity and fitness. Many children don't want to go outside to play. We need fresh ideas to reach these kids, a new method of training. Traditional training methods in organized youth sports focus primarily on preparing athletes for specific game situations. Emphasis is placed on learning specific plays and strategy. Though this is a necessary part of training, it should not be the sole focus. Unfortunately, creativity, fitness, and athletic skills are no longer developed in the backyard, schoolyard, or parks. Thus, during organized practices time must be spent on developing overall movement skills in order for kids to execute properly in game situations. Doing so will make coaching more effective and rewarding, and each child's athletic experience will be more enjoyable and beneficial.

Skateboarders, snowboarders, and BMX riders have it right. These athletes focus on free-play with friends and on developing their creativity and athletic and fitness skills. They spend hours, days, sometimes years on perfecting tricks through experimenting with combinations of athletic movements. For many years the sports community looked down on these groups because of their irreverent attitude about traditional sports. Ironically, these kids are now some of the most fundamentally sound and physically fit athletes among the new generation. In their creative tricks and maneuvers they are developing all seven athletic components—agility, balance, coordination, flexibility, speed, stamina, and strength.

Our method in this book builds trust in every child's ability to advance and continue to learn using his or her own strengths. We help children challenge themselves and gauge their own progress. Our method promotes future self-learning and self-motivation, which results in continued improvement in athletic performance—while at the same time providing proactive guidance in the prevention of bad habits. We hope our book will help spark a passion and enthusiasm for your young athletes to develop a foundation of movement skills to enhance their development in the sport of their choice.

Another concern of contemporary youth in sports programs is over-specialization (playing one sport year-round), which is becoming more and more common among young athletes. Many kids focus on one sport, playing on a school team and travel teams throughout the year and going to camps during the summer. This means little rest and recovery for body parts continually used over a prolonged period of time. Combine this with the execution of the same drills over the course of a season, or over an entire year, and you have many athletes running a high risk for overuse injuries. Our athletic fitness method, by including variations of drills and many options for improving all areas of fitness, provides a way to balance activities and competitions to better develop and prepare athletes' future performance, health, and fitness. Our approach takes repeated stress off any one body part and thereby avoids many of the overuse injuries found in young athletes today.

The fundamentals of sports don't have to be boring. They don't have to feel like work. Sports and athletic development do not need to be taught the same way they have been taught for years. The most important thing to remember as you use our method in your backyard, local park, or team practice is that it's about developing every child to his or her full potential. You'll be using the latest innovative and contemporary methods, and most important, your young athletes will be having fun. In this book we provide a guide that creates meaningful, worthwhile, and measurable results for every child interested in sports. Together, let's make sports fun again while developing your youngsters into more confident, willing, and able athletes.

CHAPTER 2

Set Up the Program

Athletic fitness development programs are not something you see available in most communities or incorporated into everyday organized youth sports programs, so you may have questions about how to start creating your program. In this chapter we'll explain in detail how to start and implement your program, from setting a schedule to location and equipment needs. We'll also discuss how to make it as enjoyable and effective as possible for your participants. After reading this chapter you'll be ready to jump into the drills and activities found in the coming chapters and begin developing a program of your own.

TYPES OF PROGRAMS

One of the benefits of our training methods is that they can be implemented in two different ways in order to meet the needs of the athlete. The first method involves a parent and child working together and developing all seven athletic components at home in preparation for participation in a particular sport. A second method is to develop a community-based league training program that develops the seven athletic components. In this program there is no specific sport in mind, so training involves general movements and skills that might apply in any sport.

Parent–Child Home Training

Parents can conduct training with their children in their own backyard to prepare their children for an upcoming sport season. A parent may recognize that a child is struggling with certain sport-specific skills and want to help the child become more proficient in the skills before the season begins. The parent can develop a program for the child that improves the child's overall athletic fitness while gradually incorporating the sport-specific skill that the athlete needs to work on.

Each child has different needs, so parents and children together can decide how many times per week to train and how many weeks the training sessions should last. Training could take place gradually, over the course of a year or so, as children progressively develop their skills. Conversely, training can be more intensive and packed into a shorter amount of time in order for the child to prepare for a specific sport season. A child who trains regularly will make more progress in self-competitions, and will increase athletic fitness more quickly, than a child who trains infrequently.

Let's look at a sample baseball training program. Baseball season is six weeks away, and the parent recognizes that the child is struggling with catching and batting skills. The parent decides that coordination training will help improve the child's catching and batting skills. The parent would develop a six-week program of two sessions per week that emphasizes coordination and is supplemented by a variety of drills from the other athletic components. The other components are important because athletes need to be multidimensional. One athletic fitness component (in this case, coordination) won't improve much unless the other athletic components are developed as well.

The first step is to select three eye–hand coordination drills from chapter 4. Incorporate these drills into each of the 12 training sessions to improve general eye–hand coordination. Then select two drills from the remaining chapters. Incorporate these drills into the first eight sessions to help the athlete improve in other fitness areas and to supplement his or her eye–hand coordination training. Do not incorporate both drills into the same session, though. Select only one drill per session, and alternate them every session so that each drill is done four times over eight sessions. After eight sessions, once the child begins to improve in the general drills that are not sport specific, choose one baseball-specific drill and incorporate it into the final four sessions.

To keep the athletes interested and to provide variety, each session should be no longer than 90 minutes. Each drill should last a maximum of 20 minutes per session, and athletes should warm up before the session and cool down afterward. Be sure to change the drills and competitions every session—kids enjoy new challenges and surprises. Also be sure to work on these skills without focusing on the child's deficiencies, which risks creating additional self-doubt, and ensure that the child finds the experience appealing and fun.

This method can apply to any sport. For example, athletes can focus on agility for soccer, speed for basketball, or balance for ice hockey. Regardless of the area of focus, the principles to remember are to (1) incorporate general (not sport-specific) drills throughout training for the component being targeted; (2) supplement these drills with drills and competitions from the other athletic component chapters; and (3) introduce sport-specific drills once the athlete shows improvement in the component being targeted.

League Training

An alternative to sport-specific home training is for a town or group of parents to create a league program based entirely on athletic skills and development. A "season" in this program focuses on a particular athletic skill (such as throwing), and the individual sessions employ drills and competitions from the seven component chapters (such as eye–hand coordination, agility, and speed) in order to improve that skill. An athlete's progress is measured by charting personal improvement in the competitions over the course of the season. This type of training might seem unconventional, but it increases a young athlete's interest in and attention to learning, resulting in more rapid development of skills.

We use the term *league* primarily because it describes for most people an organizational sports structure. However, unlike traditional leagues, there is no distinguishing between practices and games. An athletic development league is designed for competing with one's self rather than for competition among athletes. In contrast to what occurs in traditional sports leagues, this program tracks individual progress in an athlete's overall athletic skills and fundamentals. Not unlike what happens in skateboarding or snowboarding, this approach encourages kids to work on athletic fundamentals through performing and perfecting specific athletic skills. The key objectives here are that all athletes improve their athletic performance, learn something new at their own pace, and achieve high results under minimal pressure.

Also unlike on traditional teams, a coach does not have a designated team or set a starting lineup. All athletes participate equally, and every volunteer coach works with every athlete. A coach in this league is a teacher of skills, a motivator through positive reinforcement, and a keen observer.

An easy way to launch an athletic fitness program in your community is to schedule a season of two sessions—the equivalent of practices in a traditional sport league—per week over a five-week period during the off-season of a popular team sport. For example, early spring, just prior to baseball and soccer seasons, works well, as does late summer prior to fall sports, or possibly winter, depending on access to indoor facilities or weather considerations. The advantage of conducting training sessions at these times is that kids will be freshly exposed to movement training, preparing them just before their athletic season. If a child is registered to play multiple sports, or if he or she plays and specializes in the same sport over the course of the year, we highly recommend that you incorporate athletic fitness training into preseason prep and in-season practices. The drills and activities in this book are designed to be used at any time of the year, either in or out of a particular sport's season. Because drills and competitions are based on basic athletic components that form the foundation of all sports, it's advisable to use the material in this book throughout the year to obtain optimal performance results.

The season should be designed in its entirety before any child begins to participate. Coaches should plan which athletic components to include in each session and choose drills and competitions that will help the athletes improve their performances in those areas. Be sure to change the drills and competitions every session—kids enjoy new challenges and surprises. We suggest employing drills from only four different athletic components each session, but you should provide training in all seven components over the course of the program. Planning ahead allows an organized and well thought-out approach to what each young athlete will focus on and attempt to improve on. Backup drills and competitions are held in reserve in case a coach needs to make adjustments. Before the launch of each season, the goals of the season are presented to athletes and parents. Athletes should be encouraged to perform the drills and self-measuring competitions at home between sessions to increase their improvement.

Coaches should set up one station for each athletic component practiced during the session. For example, if a session focuses on coordination, balance, speed, and agility, the coaches would set up four stations. At each station, athletes will execute two to four drills with self-measuring competitions, rotating from one station to the next over the course of the session. An average session runs about 90 minutes. Coaches should allot about 20 minutes to each component station, including 5 minutes of instruction and demonstration, 5 minutes of drill work, and then 10 minutes of competitions. Coaches should also provide a 3-minute break between each station. Training should be fast paced and engaging, with no standing around. Nothing loses a kid's attention faster than inactivity.

An important component in providing an optimal environment for training is the number of volunteers you have working with you to conduct each session. Any number of athletes can participate as long as there's at least one coach or supervisor for every six athletes. This allows each child to get individual attention and observation and permits everyone equal repetitions and competition time. One coach is assigned to each station. Every volunteer must have a complete understanding of how his or her station must function in order to conduct each drill and competition and ensure that each child receives the best experience.

At the conclusion of each session, tally up the total number of self-competition points accumulated by each athlete for the four stations. This scoring method doesn't necessarily reward the athlete with the best overall performance in comparison to others; rather, it recognizes athletes who achieve the most improvement according to their ability level. We believe this is the only fair way to keep kids engaged, competitive, and rewarded, while also allowing them to advance at their own pace. We all know that young athletes progress at different paces and stages, and we want a fair way to keep all kids active and interested in athletic fitness for life.

LOCATION AND EQUIPMENT

Once you decide when to launch your athletic fitness program, you need to select a location that allows an ideal environment for training sessions to take place. An outdoor location is best since it allows more space for unrestricted movement. For home-based training, the child can perform the drills and competitions right in the backyard. A league will require significantly more space. The best outdoor location for a group of 20 to 40 kids should be about 40 yards long by 40 yards wide

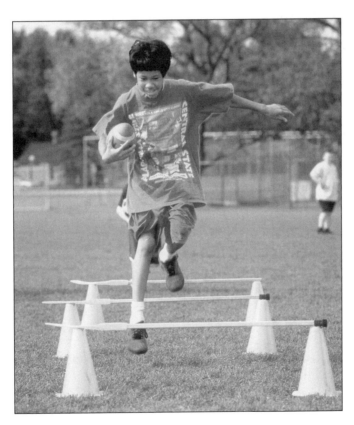

Having a location and equipment that meet the athlete's needs will make each session fun, engaging, and rewarding.

and have a flat surface of grass or turf. Access to a hard court or driveway surface that is about 15 by 15 yards or larger and access to a hill with a gradual grade is also beneficial as it provides variation. Note that these are only suggestions; we recognize that everyone is faced with different situations depending on where they live. With this in mind, we have included in every chapter drills that can be conducted in small areas and on a variety of surfaces, allowing you the opportunity and flexibility to use the drills and adjust them to meet your needs while maintaining their basic fundamentals.

Equipment is also essential to making your program effective and engaging. To make learning the fundamentals of the seven vital components in sports both contemporary and fun, we recommend that you use a combination of traditional and nontraditional equipment. The nontraditional equipment listed and used throughout the book will be items that you most likely either have not purchased in the past or did not purchase for the purpose of athletic training. Though some of this equipment can be considered athletic (specialty balls and balance items), such tools are not typically used by parents or youth coaches. For example, innovative to our athletic fitness training model is the use of video games. When dealing with kids who are continually exposed to the newest technology that ultimately leads to more sedentary activities, we have discovered that an "if you can't beat them, join them" strategy makes the most sense. Rather than fight technology, it's smarter to use it instead. Kids are so tuned in to playing video games and visually adept to learning that using these games to aid in athletic development can be a distinct advantage. Look for further explanation of the benefits of incorporating video games into practice in chapter 4.

Most traditional equipment can be purchased at any sporting goods store or major department chain and consists of the following:

Balls: baseball (hard and soft—foam or Wiffle); football (hard and soft); soccer (regulation size 4); basketball (regulation size for juniors); golf (plastic); tennis

Baseball bat (wooden and plastic)

Baseball glove (age and size appropriate)

Tennis racket

Lacrosse stick

Pitch back or rebounder (a tightly strung apparatus that returns thrown balls toward the thrower)

Measuring tape

Stopwatch

BMX or mountain bike

The following set of equipment is less standard but still used frequently by coaches in athletic training. You can easily find this equipment in catalogs or on the Web.

- Elastic tubing and bungee cords (used primarily for flexibility and strength training)
- Minihurdles (6 inch and 12 inch)
- Agility ladder
- Agility ball
- Tumbling mat (five to six feet long by three to four feet wide)
- Cones and dots (cones can be found in sporting goods and major department stores; dots are available through specialty catalogs and Web sites)
- Stackable steps (plastic stackable steps used primarily for jumping and strength training)
- Medicine ball (8- to 10-year-olds: 4-pound ball; 11- to 12-year-olds: 4-pound to 6-pound ball; 13- to 14-year-olds: 4-pound to 8-pound ball). Note that ages and weights are suggestions; common sense and size and strength of the athletes should be considered—always err on the lighter side.

The following set of equipment can be considered nontraditional because it's not widely used in athletic training. You can search for these items online or at a local store.

- Balance pods
- Vew-Do zone balance pro board
- Versa balance beam or an eight-foot two-by-four
- Reaction/agility balls
- Video game devices and games: Play Station Portable (PSP); EA Sports NFL Street; Madden NFL Football; MVP Baseball; Tiger Woods PGA Golf; NBA Street; World Cup Soccer

The equipment should be fully set up before athletes begin the session. In a league setting, there should be enough equipment to accommodate six athletes at each station. A consistent setup should be maintained, such as when a skateboarder arrives at a skate park he or she finds familiar areas of the park that never change. If you are using the same space every session, place each of the four component stations in their own space on the field in the same spot each session. Each station should have enough space to accommodate an appropriate number of separate competitions.

MAKING YOUR PROGRAM SUCCESSFUL

Your program, whether home or league based, will be successful if kids enjoy the experience. Athletic component training creates the optimal environment for natural and sensory learning. Why is experiential learning so important? Primarily because kids are often taught through command instruction—"do this" and "do that"—or have fundamentals explained to them mainly verbally, maybe with a brief demonstration (which is risky if the demo is done incorrectly), and are then expected to comprehend and execute. As a result, optimal learning doesn't take place, and kids don't fully understand how to do what's being asked of them. Allow athletes time to experiment with particular movements and techniques, with limited instruction, numerous repetitions, and instructors who assist in self-correction and give positive reinforcement to make the learning curve faster.

For example, if you're conducting a speed drill that emphasizes multiple directions (e.g., sprint 20 yards upfield; immediately stop at a designated spot; cut 45 degrees to the left and sprint 20 yards), rather than taking your athletes through each phase and technique of the drill (which takes up time and is proven to be less effective), have them carefully observe someone demonstrating the overall drill twice. Request that each athlete focus on the demonstrator's footwork only. Then have the athletes attempt the drill. If one or more of them is not cutting hard with the left foot, have the entire group run through the drill several more times, focusing only on the left foot. If they remain slow to respond to the correction, demonstrate the skill twice more, telling each athlete to focus only on the left foot at the time of the hard cut. The type of success this type of training produces encourages athletes to continue to work on the drills because they feel empowered to self-learn and correct themselves through sensory training. This is far better than an overload of verbal demands that are often not well understood.

The other important component of successful learning is self-measurement. Give the athletes chances to measure and evaluate themselves and their progress. During the season, conduct competition-only sessions at the middle and end of your program so that all athletes can measure their progress from previous sessions. Time, distance, and accuracy are the three main scoring elements in the competitions, and most of the time these measurements will indicate how well athletes can execute a drill. Success in all competitions is based on the individual. The primary objective of competitions is to self-measure progress and challenge athletes to improve their overall scores over time. Athletes may move to the next progression and competition when they feel comfortable that they're improving and can handle more advanced work. Ultimately, the self-scoring method accurately indicates if they're ready to advance. In many cases, a score of 70 percent or higher suggests that an athlete can move on to the next progression and competition. However, some individuals have difficulty reaching the 70 percent mark. As a coach or parent, use your own judgment; if athletes are consistently improving and coming close to scoring 70 percent, it's often best to allow them to advance.

Now that you're familiar with athletic fitness programs and understand the basic tenets of establishing such a program of your own, move on to the drills and begin considering which ones will work best for you and your group of young athletes. And most importantly, have fun!

Improve Flexibility

Flexibility refers to the ability to bend and move easily without injury or damage. Flexibility of muscles and ligaments is integral to overall athletic fitness because it improves range of motion, allowing an athlete to throw, kick, jump, run, or swing with more strength, power, and speed. Athletes who lack flexibility tend to have an increased risk of injury and a decreased ability to execute fundamental athletic movements, thereby compromising their overall performance. Athletes who have flexibility tend to perform basic athletic functions and skills better than those who lack it.

Flexibility plays an important role in many aspects of sport. Flexibility allows shortstops to bend and stretch in the many ways required to field ground balls. Flexibility enables soccer players to reach and gain control of balls passed to them on the ground or in the air. Flexibility allows hockey players to skate at full speed and make necessary immediate adjustments to situations as they develop on the ice. Flexibility permits basketball players to jump and reach and to control rebounds. In fact, flexibility aids nearly every athletic movement. Without flexibility, we could not become fit or execute many basic sport techniques.

During childhood, most physically active kids develop the flexibility they need naturally. That said, early flexibility training helps young athletes develop good habits that will benefit them once they reach adolescence. It's a good idea to begin flexibility drills when children are younger and have a relatively easy time executing them. During their teenage years, kids begin to lose their natural flexibility and have a more difficult time with beginning flexibility training.

In addition to the drills presented in this chapter, flexibility training is incorporated naturally into the other chapters in the book. Although this aspect of fitness is often overlooked and not given the single focus that the other six athletic components receive, when flexibility becomes part of an athlete's overall training regimen, he or she has an optimal opportunity to enhance performance. Without flexibility, athletes cannot reach their full potential in any area of athletic fitness. For example, when training athletes to improve in their movements for any field or court sport, you would not place a singular focus on linear speed and movement. Rather, you would spend time on multiple-direction speed and agility, with flexibility being integral to the athlete's successful execution of the skill. The suppleness required to efficiently stop, go, and change direction is enhanced through flexibility training.

The three main stages in which flexibility is included in youth athletics are the initial warm-up, the increase in overall range of motion, and the cool-down. Let's look at each of these stages in detail.

WARMING UP

Before the start of any practice, game, or activity that involves athletic movement, it's important to slowly heat the body up and begin to generate energy throughout the muscles. This is done by getting blood circulating to all the major muscle groups. Generally kids arrive at a practice or game after either sitting around all day or just getting out of bed in the morning. A proper warm-up before activity allows muscles to wake up and get ready for movement. Warming up is also a great way to get athletes quickly into the right state of mind for the start of an activity, practice, or game. In addition, a proper warm-up assists in the prevention of injuries by working out the stiffness that might have occurred throughout the day or overnight.

When they hear the phrase "warming up," many people think of stretching, but this is incorrect and outdated. In fact, athletes should not begin stretching before they have adequately warmed up. To begin to increase flexibility, athletes must first get their circulation flowing throughout their bodies by raising body temperature. The warm-up should begin with an emphasis on large muscle groups (thighs, hips,

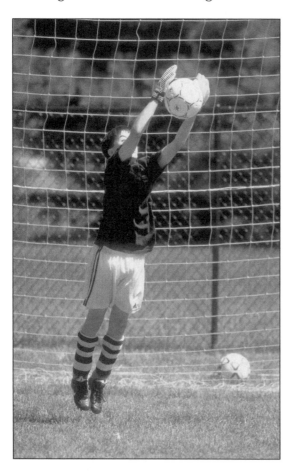

Flexibility aids nearly every athletic movement and is integral to an athlete's successful execution of skills such as reaching and jumping.

back, and shoulders) followed by a progression to the smaller muscle groups specific to the sport or activity about to occur. The focus is on the larger muscle groups at first because they require more energy to warm up. The initial period of warming up should run no longer than 8 to 10 minutes. When done properly—with limited time standing around—there's usually no need to extend a warm-up beyond 10 minutes. You don't want to tire athletes before the actual activity begins.

You want to gain your athletes' interest from the start, so the warm-up period should be fun. If your athletes seem sluggish or stubborn about warming up, try disguising the warm-up routine. For instance, you might design creative obstacle courses that are a little different each time. By changing the looks of your warm-up routine, you'll help your kids look forward to new challenges, which keeps things from getting stale. The obstacle course should emphasize the large muscle groups and is best used as the first activity in a warm-up because it immediately engages athletes and starts the training session on a positive note. When designing your obstacle course, try to incorporate all the following movements.

• **Stepping over.** These movements energize the thighs and hip flexors. You'll need an agility ladder, hurdles 6 inches and 12 inches high (six of each), or bleacher stairs. Laid flat on the ground, the agility ladder is used to get your athletes' legs moving. Athletes place each foot quickly into every space as they progress "up" the ladder. The 6-inch and 12-inch hurdles are set up about three feet apart for athletes to leap over, with the front leg driving forward. If low hurdles aren't available, set up your obstacle course close to a set of bleacher stairs. Climbing stairs replicates the movement you want. Be sure that athletes drive each leg forward when climbing the stairs or leaping over the hurdles.

• **Moving laterally.** Moving side to side replicates athletic movement, stretches out the groin, and loosens the ankles. Again, use an agility ladder, this time having kids execute lateral movements from left to right and then right to left, placing one foot in each square of the ladder. You might eventually add a tennis ball, basketball, or baseball and ask athletes to toss the ball back and forth as they move through the ladder. You might also use agility balls (odd-shaped balls with six knobs that make balls bounce in unpredictable directions) to add fun and an extra challenge once kids start to find this segment of the obstacle course too easy. The erratic bounces of the balls keep athletes on their toes as they try to catch balls bounced to them as they move across the ladder.

• **Moving low and under.** Remember that the reason you incorporate a warm-up at the start of a workout, practice, or game is to wake up the major muscle groups and get the circulation flowing to these areas; you want these muscles to be prepared to perform when called on in a particular drill or activity. Low-and-under movements get thighs, back, hip flexors, and shoulder muscles firing. If available, include four to six adjustable track hurdles in your obstacle course. Instead of using these hurdles for leaping over, use them to make athletes bend and go under. If hurdles are unavailable, have someone hold a rope or stick at varying heights for athletes to pass under.

• **Jumping.** Jumps energize the ankles, hip flexors, and thighs. Use six-inch hurdles set up about three feet apart in a straight line. Athletes perform consecutive jumps with both feet landing simultaneously. Each time the feet hit the ground, athletes immediately jump, without stopping, over the next hurdle until they have jumped over all six. Watch closely and remind athletes to land and explode off the balls of their feet.

• **Running.** A run gets the blood flowing to the heart and muscles. Traditionally a warm-up includes running for an extended period of time or conducting a series of short wind sprints. Because running is an overused warm-up technique, incorporate a fun chasing element as part of the obstacle course. Place three Frisbees at one area of the course that has about 30 yards of open space in which six athletes can run. As athletes go through the obstacle course in assigned pairs and arrive at this station, one partner (A) takes a Frisbee and tosses it downfield. The other partner (B) chases and attempts to catch the Frisbee before it hits the ground, while A also runs downfield 30 yards and waits for B to catch or retrieve the Frisbee and toss it upfield for A to catch or retrieve. Both athletes end at the original spot where the exercise began and repeat it twice before continuing to the next obstacle course element.

• **Tossing.** Tosses engage and loosen the shoulder, abdominal, and hip muscles. Tossing is best executed with a two-pound medicine ball for 8- and 9-year-olds or a four-pound medicine ball for 10- to 14-year-olds. Partners stand about nine feet apart from one another. Athletes gently toss the ball back and forth three times with both hands, similar to a basketball push-pass. They then toss the ball back and forth another three times using an overhead pass (the ball is placed behind the head and thrown gently while taking one step toward the partner and extending the arms), followed by three underhand tosses (starting from between the legs), and concluding with two tosses from each side of the body to the partner (stand with right side of the body facing partner, arms extended back; take a short step toward partner and toss the ball; repeat on the other side) before moving to the next obstacle element.

• **Tumbling and rolling.** Tumbling helps athletes become more aware of their bodies and their control. On a tumbling mat or soft surface about six to eight feet in length, have each athlete perform one forward tumble and then immediately get to the feet and sprint five yards to a cone on the right. The athlete then returns to the mat and repeats, this time running to a cone five yards away on the left. Repeat again with athletes rolling on their right sides down the mat, getting to their feet, and sprinting to the cone on their right, and then rolling on their left sides and sprinting to the cone on their left.

Obstacle courses are effective warm-ups for any sport. Execute each warm-up session as a course that they must complete three times at a comfortable pace. Remember that the objective is not to tire them out but to energize them, increase their overall flexibility, and warm up their muscles by getting their blood flowing. See page 23 for a suggested obstacle course warm-up.

After warming up the large muscles, athletes in any sport should also do a sport-specific warm-up. This warm-up, though often overlooked, is vital to an athlete's performance. If an athlete begins a training session or competition by immediately executing skills and techniques without first introducing the body to the movements that make up the skill or technique, risk of injury increases and overall movement potential is compromised.

During the sport-specific warm-up, athletes prepare for a game or practice by replicating the movements they'll be performing on the field. For example, during a baseball warm-up, outfielders should perform a routine that mimics all the movements that might occur in the outfield. The first step and pivot to turn for a fly ball over the head (to both the left and right as well as straight back) should be first walked through, then jogged, and then run at both half- and full speed. These drills should be done first without a ball and then with a ball. Then athletes should progress to repeating all drills and adding a throw to finish the play. See pages 35 to 37 for additional sport-specific warm-ups.

INCREASING RANGE OF MOTION

The main purpose of improving flexibility is to increase the athlete's range of motion (ROM). Most younger kids have fairly good ROM. As they approach puberty, they begin to experience more rapid muscular growth, and with muscle growth comes more bulk. This increased mass tends to naturally contract and tighten after and between every workout. The closer an athlete gets to the age of 12, the more emphasis that should be paid to isolated range-of-motion training to keep muscles flexible.

Without full ROM, athletes can't maximize their functional strength in throwing, kicking, jumping, running, and so on because if they can't fully extend a muscle or muscle group, less power can be generated. When athletes lack full ROM, they tend to rely on other muscle groups, which tires them faster and places undue stress on surrounding body parts. For example, if tennis players don't have adequate ROM in their shoulders, they might depend too much on their elbows and thereby cause an injury.

To maximize performance and reduce injuries, athletes should focus on increasing full ROM in two key areas, particularly: the shoulder region (including the upper back and spine) and the hip flexor region (including the buttocks and lower back). These regions are two main focal points for most sports because of the power they generate to execute many athletic tasks. When developing ROM for the shoulder area, we strongly suggest developing the entire deltoid or shoulder (front, middle, and back) along with the surrounding muscle groups of the upper back and chest areas. Hip flexors are the muscles located on each side of the lower torso, just below the waistline. The hip flexor muscle and buttocks area are important to the generation of speed and strength and also affect stamina. Developing full ROM in this area helps athletes generate power and speed. See pages 24 to 29 for ROM exercises. Note that it's important to ask athletes where they "feel the stretch," because this tells you if the exercise is affecting the intended target area.

COOLING DOWN

Cooling down involves returning an athlete's heart rate to a normal resting rate. This rate varies from athlete to athlete, but the idea is to bring the pulse rate back down gradually in order for the body to begin rest and recovery. The cool-down often involves a gradual slowing down of an athlete's last activity and eventually coming to a complete resting stop. For example, runners might end their workouts by gradually slowing their pace to a near-jog and then a walk before beginning a light stretching routine. Soccer players might finish a game that involves a combination of short and fast bursts and longer sustained slower runs with a slow sustained jog to bring body temperature and pulse rate down. This would be followed by a stretching routine.

In the past many thought flexibility could be developed only through static stretching. We suggest that the only time athletes use static stretching is when cooling down. Static stretching (holding a stretch for a short length of time) is most effective at the end of a workout or game, when the body is at its highest heat capacity. The body is more pliable at this time and better prepared to be stretched and trained to extend the muscle fibers. When the body is stiff and unable to get fully involved, such as before an athlete is fully warmed up, static stretching is less efficient and might injure the athlete. Static stretching is best used for about six to eight minutes at the very end of a practice or competition. This is also a great time to talk to your athletes or team and review what they accomplished, how they felt, and what you plan to do the next time you meet. See pages 30 to 34 for static stretches to incorporate into the cool-down.

Obstacle Course Warm-Up

Age Range

8 to 14

Purpose

To prepare the body for activity by raising the internal temperature and increasing circulation to all muscle groups; to allow the body to move more freely and to remove stiffness from previous workouts or inactivity

Benefits

Athletes increase full circulation flow in order to assist their bodies in dealing with the isolated joint and muscle stress brought on by sport-specific repetitive drills and technique work.

Equipment

You'll need two agility ladders or some chalk or paint to mark out your own boxes, 12 six-inch hurdles, six 12-inch hurdles, three agility balls, six adjustable track hurdles (if available), three Frisbees, three 2-pound medicine balls and three 4-pound medicine balls, a tumbling mat or a soft grassy area, 10 cones, and a whistle.

Setup

The course we describe here can accommodate up to 42 kids. If you have more athletes, set up two courses. Seven different stations, each based on one movement found on pages 19 to 20, make up the design of our course. A maximum of six athletes can participate at each station at one time.

Execution

Place an even number of athletes at each station and let them run through the course simultaneously. Blow a whistle to begin timing each of the seven stations for a total of two minutes per station. After every two minutes the whistle blows, and everyone at one station rotates to the next station adjacent to the one they just completed. This allows all seven stations to be operational at all times and avoids standing around and watching; every athlete is engaged and moving for the full 14 minutes. It's best to have an adult volunteer assigned to each station.

Front Shoulder ROM

Age Range

8 to 14

Purpose

To increase shoulder ROM with a focus on the front of the shoulder

Benefits

Athletes improve performance by improving flexibility in the anterior part of the shoulder. This shoulder drill applies directly to all racket sports as well as to the golf swing and pitching, batting, and throwing functions.

Equipment

Each pair of athletes needs two tennis balls.

Setup

Two athletes stand directly in front of each other with one facing the back of the other.

Execution

Athlete A faces the back of athlete B with a tennis ball in each hand at arm's length behind athlete B. Athlete B stands with hands extended in front of the chest (a) before reaching behind with one arm (b), keeping chest out and feet square, securing the tennis ball from athlete A, and returning the ball to the front of the body. Repeat with the other arm. Each athlete does 10 repetitions with each arm.

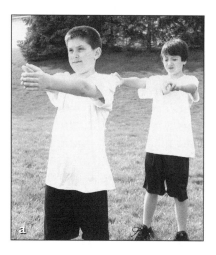
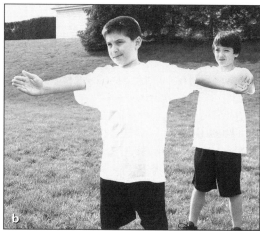

Top of Shoulder ROM

Age Range

8 to 14

Purpose

To increase shoulder ROM with a focus on the top of the shoulder

Benefits

Athletes improve performance by increasing flexibility in the top part of the shoulder. This shoulder drill directly applies to all racket sports, pitching, shooting and rebounding in basketball, volleyball, and all throwing functions.

Equipment

Each pair of athletes needs two tennis balls.

Setup

Two athletes stand directly in front of each other, one facing the back of the other.

Execution

Athlete A stands behind and faces the back of athlete B and holds one tennis ball in each hand at arm's length and shoulder-blade height behind athlete B. Athlete B stands with both hands at the sides (*a*) before reaching directly over the left shoulder with the left arm and hand (*b*), keeping the chest out and feet square, securing the tennis ball from athlete A, bringing the ball to the front and across the body and behind the left hip, and handing the ball back to athlete A. Each athlete does 10 repetitions with each arm.

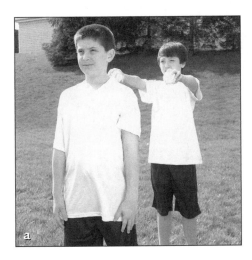
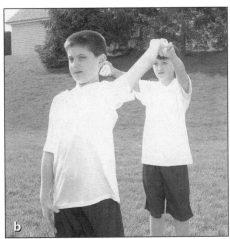

Posterior Shoulder ROM

Age Range
8 to 14

Purpose
To increase shoulder ROM with a focus on the back of the shoulder

Benefits
Athletes improve performance by increasing flexibility in the posterior part of the shoulder. This shoulder drill applies directly to all racket sports, the golf swing, batting, and backhand shots in ice hockey and lacrosse.

Equipment
Each pair of athletes needs five tennis balls.

Setup
Two athletes stand side by side about three feet apart.

Execution
Athlete A stands to the left of athlete B with a tennis ball fully extended in the left hand in front of the body. Athlete B stands with right arm fully extended from the side of the body at chest level *(a)*. Athlete B crosses the arm back across the chest and fully extends to grab the tennis ball from athlete A *(b)*. This is immediately followed by athlete B crossing the right arm with the ball back across the chest and dropping the ball when the right arm is fully extended. (Note that you might want to measure where the ball lands each time it hits the ground; the ball should land as far as possible from the athlete's body to the side.) Repeat 10 times before switching arms. Each athlete does 10 repetitions with each arm.

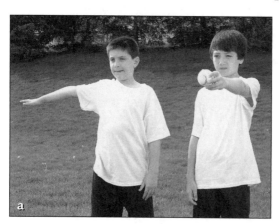
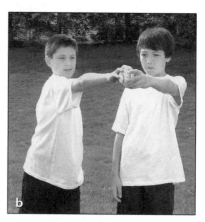

Side of Hip ROM

Age Range

8 to 14

Purpose

To increase the hips' ROM

Benefits

Athletes improve performance by increasing flexibility at the side of the hip. This drill applies directly to all kicking sports and to any sport that includes hip rotation, such as running, jumping, skating, or swinging a baseball bat, tennis racket, golf club, or hockey stick.

Equipment

A cone and some chalk

Setup

An athlete stands a few feet from a wall with one hip facing the wall.

Execution

There are two variations for each athlete to perform. The first takes the hip through a partial range of motion, and the second variation takes the hip through its full range of motion.

Cross-Body Swing

An athlete begins by swinging the left leg across the body until the ball of the foot touches the wall. Mark with a cone how far an athlete can stand away from the wall and still successfully touch the wall with the ball of the foot. Mark with chalk how high on the wall the ball of the foot touches. Repeat 10 times before switching sides for a right-hip swing. Record the distance and height from session to session to measure the progress of each athlete's flexibility.

Cross-Body Pendulum Swing

An athlete stands several feet from a wall with the right hip facing the wall. The athlete begins by swinging the left leg out to the side of the body away from the wall, as high as the leg allows *(a)*. The left leg then returns across the body (similar to a pendulum) until the left foot touches the wall *(b)*. Mark with a cone how far an athlete can stand away from the wall and still touch the wall with the ball of the foot. A partner can mark with chalk how high on the wall the ball of the left foot touches. Repeat 10 times before switching sides for a right-hip swing. Record the distance and height from session to session to measure the progress of each athlete's flexibility.

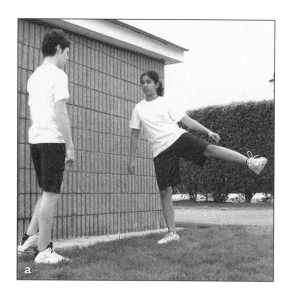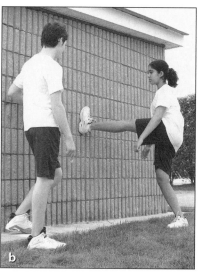

Front and Side of Hip ROM

Age Range

8 to 14

Purpose

To increase the hips' ROM

Benefits

Athletes improve athletic performance by increasing flexibility on the front and side of the hip. This drill applies to all kicking sports as well as to any sport that includes hip rotation (e.g., swinging a baseball bat, tennis racket, golf club, or hockey stick), running, jumping, or skating.

Equipment

A cone and some chalk

Setup

An athlete stands a few feet from a wall with both hips facing square to the wall.

Execution

Athletes perform forward and backward hip swings and measure their progress.

Forward Swing

From the starting position (a), each athlete begins by swinging the right leg straight up and out until the ball of the foot touches the wall (b). Mark with a cone how far each athlete can stand away from the wall and still touch the wall with the ball of the foot. Mark with chalk how high on the wall the foot touches. Repeat 10 times before switching sides for a left-leg hip swing. Record the distance and height from one session to the next to measure the progress of each athlete's flexibility.

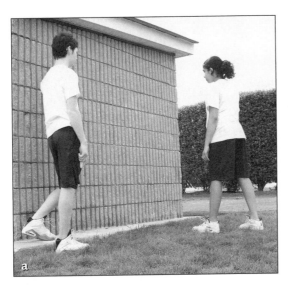 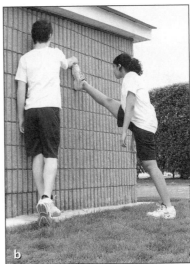

Backward Swing

Athletes stand several feet from a wall with their backs to the wall. Hips remain square to the wall. Each athlete begins by swinging the right leg straight back and up until the ball of the foot touches the wall. Mark with a cone how far they can stand away from the wall and still touch the wall with the ball of the foot. Mark with chalk how high on the wall the ball of the foot touches. Repeat 10 times before switching sides for a left-leg hip swing. Record the distance and height from session to session to measure the progress of each athlete's flexibility.

Static Stretches

Age Range

8 to 14

Purpose

To increase overall flexibility through isolated stretches

Benefits

Stretching helps prevent injuries by extending muscle fibers, and it is most effective at the end of a workout or competition.

Equipment

Strength band

Setup

Athletes spread out on flat grass or another soft surface.

Execution

Athletes execute a variety of stretches that target every major muscle group.

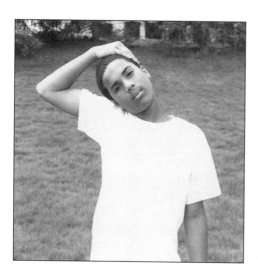

Neck

With feet flat on the ground and shoulder-width apart, an athlete takes the right hand and places it on the left side of the head just above the left ear. The athlete then gently pushs the head and neck with the right hand down toward the right shoulder. If possible, allow the right ear to touch the right shoulder, and hold for two seconds. Repeat 10 times, and then reverse the exercise to the left side.

Torso and Back

The athletes sit with straight backs, knees bent, toes pointed slightly up, and with weight on their heels *(a)*. They tuck their chins down, bend down at the hips, and pull forward and down between the knees as far as they can go *(b)*. They hold both hands on the outside of each leg and gently pull their torsos toward their feet. They hold for two seconds, release, and repeat 10 times.

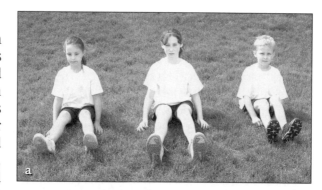

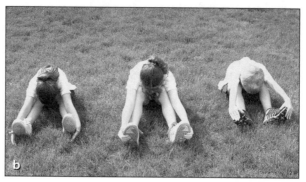

Arms and Shoulders

Athletes stand with feet shoulder-width apart and arms by each side. They then swing both arms straight up, with elbows extended and palms facing each other. They touch the fingertips of each hand and hold for two seconds. Repeat 10 times.

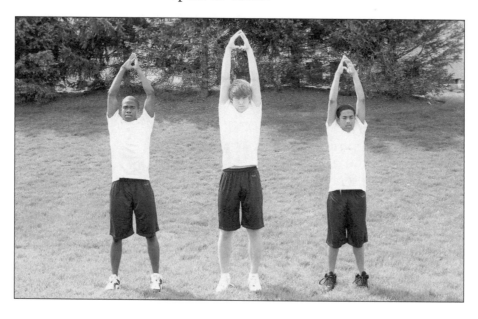

Hips and Lower Back

Athletes lie flat on their backs. Each athlete holds a strength band on both ends and places the right foot in the middle of the loop. The band wraps around the outside of the ankle and then around between the legs. Each athlete lifts the right leg with the right heel point-ing across the body toward the left side above the left leg (positioned flat on the ground); the right knee is locked. When the right leg can extend no fur-ther across the body above the left leg, the athlete gently pulls on the ends of the band to extend the stretch slightly and holds for two seconds. Repeat 10 times on each side.

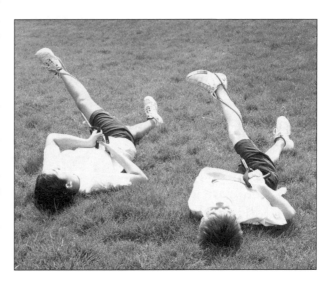

Groin

In a squatting position, the athlete stretches the left leg directly out on the left side of the body with the left heel placed on the ground, toes up, torso facing straight ahead. The majority of the body weight is balanced between the right squatting leg and the left heel. Hold for two seconds. Then reverse sides, stretch over to the opposite side, and hold for two seconds. Repeat 10 times.

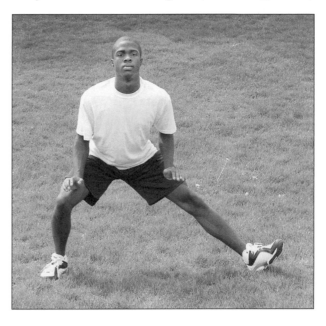

Calves and Achilles

Each athlete stands facing a pole or wall. The athlete places both hands on the pole with arms extended. The left knee is lifted off the ground, and all weight is placed on the right heel, which is flat on the ground.

Encourage athletes to lean into the stretch to maximize the extension of the right Achilles tendon and calf muscle. Hold for three seconds, and repeat 10 times. Switch and repeat 10 more times on the left Achilles and calf.

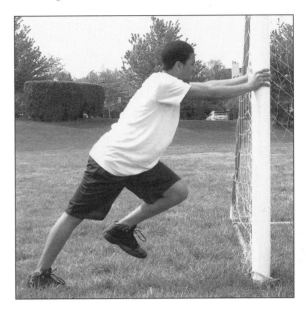

Hamstrings and Lower Back

Athletes lie flat on their backs with knees slightly bent. They slowly bring their left knees to their chests 10 times, hold for two seconds each time, and then repeat with their right knees. They continue the stretch by bringing both knees to their chests for another 10 repetitions, holding for two seconds each time.

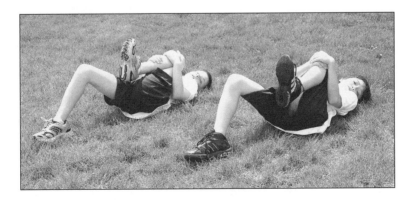

Hamstrings

Athletes lie flat on their backs with knees slightly bent. Each athlete loops a strength band around the left foot and brings the foot straight up, with the heel facing flat toward the sky, and holds for three seconds. Repeat 10 times total, and switch feet for another 10 repetitions.

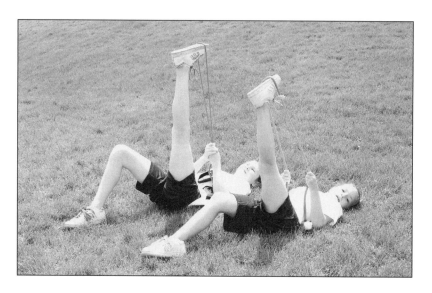

Quads

Athletes are on their hands and knees. Each athlete bends the right knee and extends it back and off the ground. The foot is brought straight up until the athlete can grasp the ankle with the right hand. The thigh should be parallel to the ground, and the back should not arch. Hold for two seconds, and repeat 10 times total before switching legs.

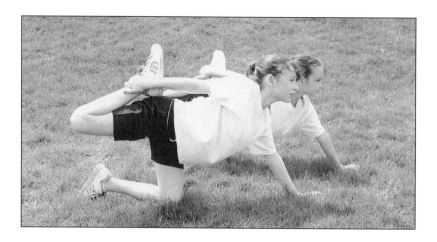

Soccer Warm-Up

Age Range

8 to 14

Purpose

To warm athletes up and prepare them for movements on the soccer field

Benefits

Athletes improve performance by replicating moves commonly used on the field of competition.

Equipment

Six soccer balls, three 6-inch hurdles, three cones

Setup

Create a warm-up course that each athlete runs through three times consecutively. The course is set up in an area 35 yards by 20 yards. As many as 18 kids can consecutively go through the course, one after the other, as long as they're careful not to run into the athlete in front of them.

Execution

Each athlete begins laterally traveling left to right and tapping three soccer balls twice each with alternating feet (using the ball of each foot). The athlete then runs 10 yards to a cone, plants the right foot,

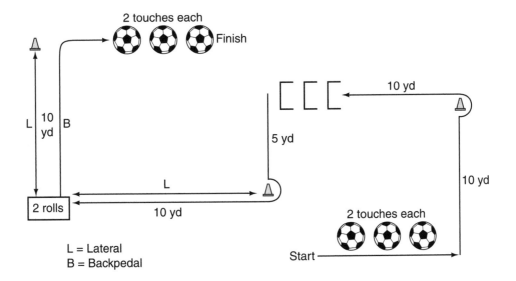

and runs another 10 yards to the left before jumping consecutively over three 6-inch hurdles. The athlete then runs 5 yards to the left, plants with the left foot (at a designated cone), runs 10 yards, rolls twice in the same direction, gets up, and runs 10 yards away from the rolling area with the left shoulder facing the rolling area and the left foot crossing over the right. At 10 yards (designated by a cone), the athlete switches over with the right shoulder facing the rolling area and the left foot crossing over the right foot for another 10 yards back to the rolling area. Then the athlete squares the hips to face the course and crosses the right foot over the left (traveling right to left), keeping the hips square for 10 yards before reversing direction back with the left foot crossing over the right (keeping hips square) 10 yards. The athlete finishes the lap by backpedaling 10 yards away from the course, stopping, and laterally traveling right to left while tapping three soccer balls twice each with alternating feet (using the ball of each foot).

Sport-
Specific
Drill

DRILL 3.9
Tennis Warm-Up

Age Range

8 to 14

Purpose

To prepare athletes for movements on the tennis court

Benefits

Athletes improve performance by replicating specific and commonly used moves on the field of competition.

Equipment

Four tennis balls, one agility ball, four cones or flat rubber dots

Setup

On half a tennis court, design a diamond shape using cones or flat rubber dots. One tennis ball is placed on the ground on each of these designated spots (marked by cones or flat dots): outside corner of the far-left service box, outside corner of the right service box, and midpoint of the baseline. A coach stands at the midpoint of the net with one agility ball and one tennis ball. One athlete runs the course at a time.

Execution

An athlete begins the warm-up on the baseline at the midpoint of the court. The athlete runs to the tennis ball placed at the corner of the left service box. A right-handed athlete bends to pick up the ball, and, without straightening to throw, executes a backhand throw (forehand for lefties) over the net. A forehand throw is a sidearm-type throw with the hand and elbow at hip level in a similar position as in a forehand tennis shot. A backhand throw, similar to a backhand tennis shot, is executed with the back of the arm facing the target and the palm of the hand twisted to face the target to release the ball. The athlete then runs to the far corner of the right service box, retrieves the ball, and, without straightening to throw, executes a forehand throw (backhand throw for lefties) over the net. The athlete then runs to the tennis ball placed at the midpoint of the baseline, and, without straightening to throw, executes a forehand toss (forehand for lefties as well), throwing the ball as far as possible over (or toward) the net. The athlete then runs immediately toward the net at its midpoint, where someone drops an agility ball as soon as the athlete crosses the service-box lines. The athlete retrieves the ball and places it at the base of the net, marked by a designated cone, and immediately begins to execute a backpedal toward the baseline. The drill concludes with the coach tossing a ball in the air over the head of the athlete during the backpedal. The athlete attempts to catch the ball with the racket hand and in one motion throw the ball over the net. Each athlete runs the course three times to complete the warm-up.

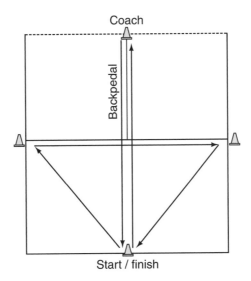

Gain Coordination

Coordination can be described as the skillful and balanced movement of different parts of the body at the same time. For our purposes in this chapter, coordination includes any isolated or combined balanced movement of the upper and lower body, the hands and eyes, and the feet and eyes. Athletes are often required to synchronize different body parts, movements, and tasks simultaneously in order to execute a play on the field, court, or ice. A good example is a wide receiver in football stretching to catch a pass while keeping one foot inbounds. This play involves synchronizing upper- and lower-body position while at the same time focusing on an eye–hand execution of catching the ball and an eye–foot element of keeping at least one foot inbounds. These eye–hand and eye–foot dynamics and how they combine with other body movements are the main elements we'll focus on in this chapter.

Some consider coordination an athlete's most essential tool. Athletes might be incredibly fit and have great speed, stamina, strength, and flexibility, but without coordination they can't execute the particulars of a sport. For example, a hockey player who can skate but can't handle a stick or take a shot while skating will not be effective on the ice. To move fluently on a field or court or on the ice, you need to develop the overall coordination of different body parts. A lacrosse player who seems to naturally maneuver around a defender by cutting one way and quickly changing direction and moving in another has coordinated various body parts to move and react without having to think about all the different elements that must take place. Such skills are developed primarily through agility training, covered in chapter 9.

Coaches should strive to improve their athletes' performances through creative coordination training. Athletes need to acquire specific coordination skills before they can learn how to catch, kick, throw, swing, and hit effectively. Eye–hand and eye–foot coordination during movement applies to all sports, so kids must become comfortable and fully aware of how their bodies move, synchronize, and respond in different situations. Athletes who fall short in fully developing their coordination will lack the sport-specific skills they need in order to succeed. All children, regardless of experience in their sport, can benefit from supplemented general and focused coordination training in addition to sport-specific

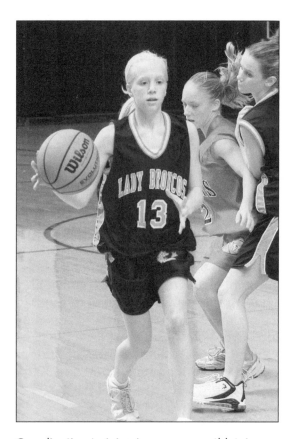

Coordination training improves an athlete's ability to synchronize upper- and lower-body position while executing at the same time an eye–hand task.

preparation. Athletes at all levels of natural ability can improve their coordination skills. Professional athletes spend countless hours training their coordination skills in order to improve their sport-specific techniques. For continued improvements to occur, coordination should be reinforced for all athletes at all levels.

Coordination involves the ability of athletes to visualize a movement in the mind and transform that visualization into motion. For success in developing coordination, athletes must first improve their overall body awareness. By continuously experiencing a movement, athletes begin to develop a feel for how that skill should be executed. As they understand how a movement should feel, athletes establish muscle memory in which the body memorizes the coordination of the movement until it becomes second nature, or automatic. Once muscle memory is established, coordination and execution of a move improves rapidly; athletes can then adjust this memory, or knowledge, to various conditions in order to execute the precise movements of a skill. For example, baseball infielders fielding a ground ball must first get into a wide stance with the two feet forming a wide base. This position allows for the athletes' rear-ends to get down as low as possible, which automatically forces their hands out in front of their bodies, creating a triangle between the glove and two feet. Once they have assumed this position, ask players to imagine picking up something in front of them. After several repetitions, place a baseball several feet in front of each player and ask them to repeat the wide stance and squat while reaching toward the ball. This is the position players must be in when fielding any type of ground ball that they can get in front of. This kind of exercise creates muscle memory, allowing athletes to automatically remember, through feel, how to get into proper position to execute plays. Because they don't have to think, they can react more quickly and with self-confidence when they face similar situations during competition.

Learning occurs best when kids are given opportunities to experience and feel the movement of a skill. Formal cognitive instruction is seldom enough by itself and is sometimes overdone. Lengthy and detailed explanations of how to perform a skill can be detrimental because they can spoil the body's natural ability to execute. We have all taught ourselves difficult physical tasks through experience and trial and error. We began with crawling, progressed to walking, and eventually moved to such skills as riding a bicycle. We might have needed no instruction or any sort of lesson. We learned difficult coordination tasks on our own by experimenting and experiencing movements. The coordination drills we introduce and employ in this book won't include lengthy explanations that you must pass on to your athletes. We have designed these drills to be developed through experiential self-learning and measuring methods, which involve many repetitions. In experiential learning, athletes find their own customized ways to execute while focusing on key fundamentals. They self-correct based on feel. Thus, the drills in this chapter allow coaches to provide guided exploration and discovery for their athletes without a lot of verbal instruction. This saves you time and encourages athletes to self-learn—with support, as needed.

Along with experience, imitation is also a powerful learning tool. Humans, especially children, are hard-wired for imitation. Recently, scientists have begun to speculate that mirror neurons in the brain, which can be triggered by both seeing and performing the same activity, may allow us to train our physical movements based on pure observation. (For a discussion of this topic, see Clive Thompson's article "The Home-Screen Advantage" in the June, 2006, issue of the *New York Times Sports Magazine*.) In other words, through watching others perform a skill, athletes might subconsciously learn the skill being observed.

Coaches and athletes have long used imagery, such as videos and observation of others, to perfect skills. When it comes to coordinating and perfecting combinations of body movements, we also suggest using sport video games to stimulate the brain's neurons. Sport video games are now so sophisticated and based on such precise player movements and execution that the need for actual video is no longer necessary. You can now use portable handheld video consoles, such as the Sony PSP, to observe athletic movement and execution. Consider how passionate many kids are about playing video games. Take advantage of this contemporary approach to instruction. We recommend bringing a PSP outside to supplement the drills in this chapter by allowing the athlete to observe the execution of specific drills in virtual reality.

Video games might also help athletes develop eye–hand coordination. Studies by James Rosser of Beth Israel Deaconess Medical Center in New York have shown that surgeons who prepped for surgical drills by first playing video games for 20 minutes performed the drills 20 minutes faster and with fewer errors than those who did not play the video games. (To read more, see Michael Marriott's article, "We Have to Operate, but Let's Play First," in the February 4, 2005, issue of the *New York Times*.) Playing video games sharpens coordination, reaction time, and visual skills—all essential elements that are incorporated into the drills in this chapter.

Remember that it's important not to complicate the process of learning a skill. Many kids get stressed about what they must remember to do every time they're about to execute a skill. Athletes must learn to focus on one particular element of a skill and allow their bodies to naturally take over the other aspects. This singular focus exercise allows them to relax and focus on the feel of the skill without the pressure of attempting to decipher multiple aspects of execution. In this chapter we provide fun competitions in which kids can begin to experiment with coordination skills while focusing on only one aspect of the skill being executed. Note that coordination plays a key role in the development of many of the other athletic components that an athlete must work to develop, such as agility, balance, speed, and strength. The four chapters that feature these physical qualities also incorporate coordination elements in drills and competitions by emphasizing the coordination of multiple and simultaneous body movements.

Regardless of whether an athlete is attempting to dribble a soccer ball or basketball, stick-handle a puck or lacrosse ball, or hit a tennis ball while running full speed, the movements involved require synchronization of several body parts while in motion. The drills that follow are aimed at improving overall and specific coordination skills, which will in turn improve the fundamentals and elements of specific sports skills such as hitting a baseball or tennis ball, catching a ball while avoiding a defender, or dribbling a soccer ball while reacting to teammates and defenders on the field.

DRILL 4.1
Stomp and Clap

Age Range

8 to 14

Purpose

To develop coordination in the lower body, the upper body, and in combination through three progressions

Benefits

Athletes begin to develop mind and body awareness of specific movements and extremities while in motion. Many sports require the upper and lower body to be engaged at the same time but focused on different tasks, such as a first baseman catching a baseball while finding and tagging first base with his or her foot.

Equipment

Four cones

Setup

Four cones designate a 20-yard length of space; width is determined by the number of athletes participating at one time. Athletes should have at least an arm's length of space between them.

Execution

There are three progressions. Athletes begin by simply walking and coordinating the movement of each foot, then progress to incorporating the upper body and arms, and then finish with a combination of using both legs and arms.

Progression 1

While walking, athletes lift and stomp their left feet after three steps followed by their right feet after three steps; they continue, alternating feet every third step for 20 yards.

Progression 2

While walking, athletes clap hands on every third step for 20 yards.

Progression 3

While walking, athletes clap hands and stomp, alternating feet on every third step for 20 yards.

Reactive Knee Lifts

Age Range

8 to 14

Purpose

To develop coordination in the lower body through the use of two progressions

Benefits

Athletes begin to develop mind and body awareness of specific movements and extremities while in motion. Such an awareness might benefit soccer players, for example, who often find themselves running downfield and having to suddenly leap over a defender's legs to avoid being tackled and taken out of the play.

Equipment

Six cones

Setup

Six cones designate areas 20 and 30 yards long; width is determined by the number of athletes participating. Athletes should have at least an arm's length of space between them.

Execution

There are two progressions. Begin with walking while coordinating the movement of each leg and progress to jogging with the same coordination.

Progression 1

While walking *(a)*, athletes alternate lifting one knee every three steps, starting with the left knee *(b)*, for 20 yards. They then return and repeat one time. Each lift should be quick and exaggerated upward toward the chest.

Progression 2

While jogging, athletes alternate lifting one knee every third stride, starting with the right leg, for 30 yards, then return and repeat one time. Each lift should be quick and exaggerated upward toward the chest.

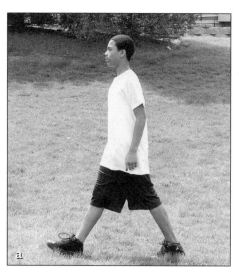 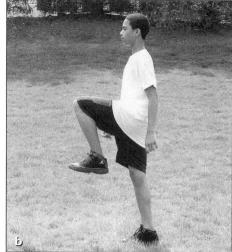

Multidirectional Lunges

Age Range

8 to 14

Purpose

To develop coordination in the lower body through the use of two progressions

Benefits

Athletes begin to develop mind and body awareness of specific movements of extremities while in motion. This is helpful in ice hockey, for example, in which players are often required to react to multiple situations and conditions while skating on the ice, such as lunging to gain control of the puck or being knocked off balance while chasing.

Equipment

Four cones

Setup

Four cones designate an area 20 yards long; width is determined by the number of athletes participating at one time. Athletes should have at least an arm's length amount of space between them.

Execution

There are two progressions. Begin with athletes walking and coordinating the lunge movement of each leg, and progress to a change in direction that accounts for variables while in motion. A lunge is executed by lowering the hips toward the ground by squatting with

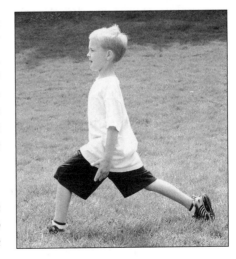

the front leg stepping out with the knee bent (keeping back straight and erect) while the back leg extends back with body weight on the ball of the foot and the knee approaching the ground. Athletes drive up from the lunge with the front foot into two steps on the balls of the feet to perform a lunge with the opposite leg.

Progression 1

Each athlete walks into a lunge using the left leg, followed by two small light steps on the balls of the feet, and then lunges using the right leg. The athlete then repeats, alternating leg lunges for 20 yards. Athletes should complete one full walk back and forth for a total of 40 yards.

Progression 2

Athletes start by jogging in place. On a signal, each athlete lunges with the left leg to a 10 o'clock position two consecutive times *(a)*. This is followed by immediately lunging with the right leg to a 2 o'clock position *(b)*. The athlete continues by lunging to the left with the left leg to the 10 o'clock position once and then immediately once to the right with the right leg to the 2 o'clock position. Each athlete begins running in place again, and repeats the entire sequence five times.

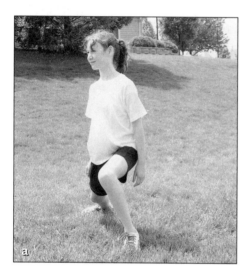 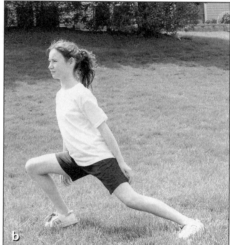

DRILL 4.4
Coordinated Skips

Age Range

8 to 14

Purpose

To develop coordination in the lower body through the use of two progressions

Benefits

Athletes begin to develop mind and body awareness of specific movements and lower extremities while in motion. Soccer players, who often find themselves running downfield and having to change their pace or direction suddenly to field a ball, are among the many athletes who might benefit from increased mind and body awareness.

Equipment

Six cones

Setup

Six cones designate areas 20 yards and 30 yards long; the number of athletes participating at one time determines the area's width. Athletes should have at least an arm's length of space between them.

Execution

There are two progressions. Athletes begin walking while adding a skip step. A skip step is a simple leap in which the lead foot gently leaves the ground slightly and skips forward for one stride.

Progression 1

While walking, the athlete executes a skip step on every third step for 20 yards.

Progression 2

While jogging lightly, the athlete executes a skip step every third stride for 30 yards.

Eye–Foot Coordination

Age Range

8 to 14

Purpose

To improve eye–foot coordination through four progressions

Benefits

Athletes perform a series of techniques that improve kicking stationary and moving balls for accuracy, distance, and power. Kicking a stationary ball can be difficult for younger athletes, and when the ball is moving, the kick becomes even more of a challenge. Eye–foot coordination is important in several sports, particularly in soccer and football.

Equipment

Each athlete needs three 8.5 × 11 inch velvet craft sheets (one black or blue, one green, and one red) with peel-off adhesive backing. The sheets are cut into 2-inch circles (three circles red, three circles green, two circles black or blue). You can find velvet craft sheets in any craft specialty store. You'll also need two soccer balls of two different colors. Use size 4 balls for 8- to 12-year-olds and size 5 balls for 13- and 14-year-olds. Four 12-inch hurdles are used for goals.

Setup

You'll need a 10×10 yard space for each athlete.

Execution

There are four progressions. Begin with a simple eye–foot coordination exercise that teaches the eye and foot to identify and then immediately execute. Athletes move to the next progression once they can correctly identify the colors on the ball facing them and can execute solid contact with the correct areas of the kicking foot. We recommend that athletes advance to the next progression in all of these drills and competitions once they have achieved a 70 percent success rate. The second progression and competition adds the dynamic of a moving ball that must be identified correctly and then kicked correctly with the proper area of the foot. Athletes must also select the correct direction to kick toward (to their right or left) and aim to kick for accuracy through a goal that's 12 inches high. The third progression reduces the total number of elements to be executed but adds the dynamic of two moving objects that must be identified and coordinated with the foot and eyes. The fourth progression and competition includes identifying the two moving soccer balls but adds the elements of fast-thinking accuracy at multiple targets (four stationary 12-inch goals).

Progression 1

Tape a two-inch color dot (black or blue) on the instep of each foot. Place six two-inch dots (three green, three red) at equal distances on a soccer ball, green on one side and red on the other. Begin by spinning the ball on the ground in front of the athlete. The athlete calls out the correct color that ends up facing him or her when the ball comes to a stop and then as quickly as possible kicks the ball. The athlete must try to call out and kick at the very moment the ball stops spinning. Ball contact occurs at the site of the two-inch dot taped onto the instep of the shoe. Be sure athletes can execute this drill successfully with both feet.

Progression 2

A ball is rolled toward the athlete from six yards away. The athlete must call out the correct color and kick the ball through one of the two 12-inch goals placed five yards away to the right and to the left of the athlete. Which goal the athlete must aim for may be called out by a partner (e.g., the partner might yell "left goal!"). The ath-

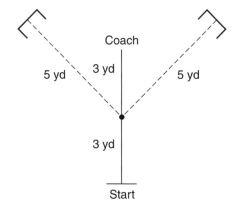

lete must use the side of the foot or the instep (directly on the shoe-laces), marked by either a black or blue circle stuck to the shoes.

Competition

Each athlete executes the drill 10 times (five kicks with the right foot and five with the left foot), earning a point each time he or she successfully calls the correct color, another point for using the correct areas of the foot to kick, and another point for kicking the ball through the proper goal. The maximum number of points that can be earned is 30.

Progression 3

A partner stands 10 yards from the athlete and rolls simultaneously two different color soccer balls directly at the athlete. The athlete begins running toward the balls as soon as they are released. When the partner calls out a color, the athlete must correctly and accurately kick the correct color ball back to the partner.

Competition

Each athlete executes the drill 10 times (five times with the right foot and five with the left), earning a point each time he or she kicks the correct ball, another point for using the instep of the foot, and another point for delivering the ball back to the feet of the partner. The maximum number of points that can be earned is 30.

Progression 4

Four 12-inch goals are positioned in the corners of a 7 × 7 yard area. Athletes kick the correct color ball in one motion through a goal 5 yards away. A coach or partner stands 8 yards from the athlete and rolls simultaneously two different color soccer balls directly at the athlete. The athlete begins running toward the balls as soon as they are released. When the partner calls out one specific color, the athlete kicks the ball of that color through one of the four goals without stopping or hesitating during the approach to the ball. The partner rolls four sets of balls total, and the athlete must kick each ball through a different goal. Be sure the athlete kicks one set of four balls with one foot, then kicks another set of four balls with the other foot.

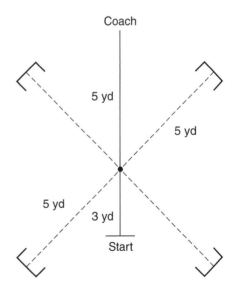

 Athletes execute two rotations for each foot, for 16 kicks total. They earn a point for every correct ball kicked and another point for every successful goal, up to a maximum of 32 points.

DRILL 4.6
■ Circle Dribbling ■

Age Range

8 to 14

Purpose

To improve eye–foot coordination and overall footwork through two progressions

Benefits

Athletes develop footwork and eye–foot coordination. Though used primarily as a soccer drill, this activity is also helpful to other sports. Athletes who are aware of how their feet move and interact with one another clearly have an advantage in competition.

Equipment

You'll need enough cones to mark off two circles and one soccer ball per athlete. If you have access to a Sony PSP, incorporate FIFA Street 2 Soccer by EA Sports into the drill. The video game shows young athletes how creative and coordinated they can be as they observe the dribbling and receiving skills of the virtual athletes in the game.

Setup

Using cones, form two circles, one about 10 yards in diameter and the other about 5 yards in diameter.

Execution

There are two progressions. Begin with a simple ball-control dribble in which athletes react to commands to execute controlling the ball with different parts of the feet. The second progression involves a smaller space in which to dribble (5 × 5 yards), and athletes must stay focused on a coach or partner making hand signals that the athletes must identify and call out.

Progression 1

Start each athlete with a soccer ball inside a circle marked off by cones (about 10 yards in diameter). Begin by having the athlete move around the circle dribbling the ball with controlled touches with different parts of the foot (inside, instep, outside, sole). Call out one specific part of the foot that can touch the ball. The athlete can use either foot to move the ball but must use only the part of the foot that has been called out. Focus on each part of the foot for 30 seconds; then the athlete rests for 60 seconds before repeating the drill with the opposite foot.

Progression 2

Repeat the drill in a smaller circle (five yards in diameter) with athletes keeping their heads up. They perform the drill by controlling the ball with the inside, outside, instep, and sole of their shoes for 30-second intervals. Every 10 seconds, have a partner hold up a different number of fingers that the athlete must identify and call out. The purpose for calling out the number of fingers is to verify that athletes have their heads up and are not looking at their feet and the ball. This helps develop foot coordination without the benefit of sight.

DRILL 4.7
Lower-Body Juggling

Age Range

8 to 14

Purpose

To improve eye–foot and lower-body coordination, overall body awareness, and control

Benefits

Athletes become better aware of how the lower body reacts and moves through a variety of situations with different movements and control. This drill is best used in soccer but can also be useful for ice hockey, football, lacrosse, or any sport in which athletes must control body movement while executing a second eye–hand or eye–foot task.

Equipment

One soccer ball per athlete

Setup

Minimal space is required, but provide enough room for athletes to feel comfortable.

Execution

There are four progressions. Athletes begin by juggling a ball on their thighs and feet. They then progress to controlling and juggling a Hacky Sack. This is followed by each athlete turning and receiving a ball to control and juggle.

Progression 1

Have each athlete take a soccer ball, drop it to the thigh, and attempt to softly transfer the ball to the other thigh. Cushioning the ball as it lands on the thigh (executed by slightly pulling back the thigh as the ball is about to land, as if attempting to catch an egg on the thigh without cracking the shell) prior to bouncing the ball several times on the one thigh before transferring it to the other thigh provides the athlete with a sense of feel and control.

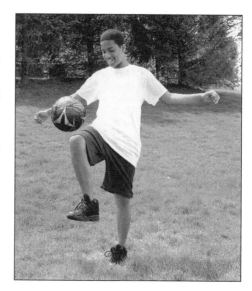

Competition

Count the number of times the athlete can successfully transfer the ball from one leg to the other without allowing the ball to drop to the ground. Success is self-measured by attempting to beat the previous or best performance.

Progression 2

Athletes repeat the previous progression but receive and transfer a soccer ball at the feet rather than the thigh. The same "catching" technique used for the thigh applies for the foot. Cushioning the ball as it lands on the foot before bouncing the ball to the other foot provides a sense of feel and control.

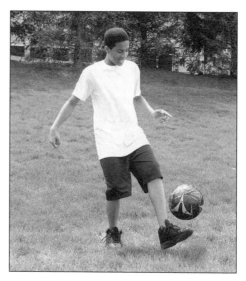

Competition

Count the number of times the ball is successfully transferred from one foot to the other without the ball dropping to the ground. Success is self-measured as athletes attempt to beat a previous or best performance.

Progression 3

Advance the drill by incorporating a Hacky Sack rather than a soccer ball and repeating the routine as described in the first two progressions. This requires adjusting to a smaller ball that takes more skill to juggle.

Progression 4

Athletes repeat the previous drill but now stand with their backs to a partner serving them a soccer ball. Once the partner verbally signals for the athlete to turn toward him or her, the partner throws the ball; the athlete must receive and control the ball on either the thigh or foot. Athletes progress by receiving the ball after the turn on the thigh or foot and continuing to juggle several times before allowing the ball to land on the ground.

Competition

Count the number of times the ball is successfully received and juggled at least three consecutive times. Count the number of times the ball is successfully transferred from one foot to the other without dropping to the ground. Success is self-measured as athletes attempt to beat a previous or best performance.

DRILL 4.8
Spot the Ball

Age Range

8 to 14

Purpose

To improve eye–hand coordination by making contact with moving objects

Benefits

Athletes improve their overall eye–hand coordination, which is important for baseball, lacrosse, tennis, ice hockey, and many other sports. This drill is not intended to improve a baseball player's hitting technique—only his or her eye–hand coordination. As we mentioned earlier, hitting a baseball can be extremely difficult. In this drill we'll focus only on contacting the ball, which is probably the most important aspect of hitting. Note that this drill provides the athlete 100 swings of the bat, an ideal experiential exercise that allows the mind to focus on one aspect (locating and identifying the ball) without other thoughts interfering.

Equipment

20 Wiffle balls, one plastic bat, 20 plastic golf balls, four permanent markers to mark each set of 20 Wiffle and plastic golf balls as follows: five balls with green dots, five balls with red dots, five balls with blue dots, and five balls with orange dots

Setup

This drill requires a 10-yard by 10-yard area, preferably against a fence so that it's easier to collect the balls.

Execution

Five progressions advance and challenge athletes to focus on the ball in order to make contact on a consistent basis.

Progression 1

Each athlete begins with a plastic bat and a Wiffle ball. Using Wiffle balls eliminates any fear of being hit by a pitched ball and allows athletes to focus full attention on making contact. A partner stands about five yards away and pitches balls overhand. Begin with athletes attempting to hit the first 20 balls pitched. They should swing at *all* balls, regardless if they are in the strike zone. The more balls you have, the better this drill works; we recommend using at least 20 Wiffle balls.

Progression 2

Batters continue to swing at every ball thrown, but now they shout out "ball!" as soon as they locate the ball leaving the pitcher's hand. This disciplines the athlete to locate the ball as early as possible and increases the success rate of hitting the ball. The key to improving eye–hand coordination is to locate and identify the ball as early as possible.

Competition

Count the number of balls hit out of 20. Tipped balls count as hits. Award 1 point for a tipped or foul ball and 2 points for all other solid contacts. Record the total number of points for every 20 pitches; the maximum number of points that can be scored is 40 for every 20 pitches. Athletes self-measure and track their personal best.

Progression 3

To increase the difficulty of identifying the ball and improve the athlete's overall focus, mark each ball with quarter-inch color dots, two per ball; mark each ball with a different color. Ask athletes to identify the color dot on the ball as soon as the ball leaves the pitcher's hand.

Competition

Count the number of balls hit out of 20. Tipped balls count as hits. Award 1 point for a tipped or foul ball, 2 points if the tipped ball is correctly identified, 3 points for all solid contacts, or 4 points for solid contact plus correct color identification. Record the number of points for every 20 pitches; the maximum number of points that can be scored is 80 for every 20 pitches. Athletes self-measure and track their personal best.

Progression 4

Advance the drill by using plastic golf balls instead of Wiffle balls. Batters continue to swing at every ball thrown and to shout out "ball!" as soon as they locate the ball leaving the pitcher's hand. Using the smaller ball disciplines the athlete and increases the success rate of hitting the regulation-size ball later. The key to improving eye–hand coordination is to locate and identify the ball as early as possible.

Competition

Count the number of balls hit out of 20. Tipped balls count as hits. Assign 1 point for a tipped or foul ball and 2 points for all other solid contacts. Record the number of points for every 20 pitches; the maximum number of points that can be scored is 40 for every 20 pitches. Athletes self-measure and track their personal best.

Progression 5

Advance the drill by incorporating 1/8-inch color dots on the plastic golf balls. Use a different color on each ball and three dots per ball. Batters continue to swing at every pitched ball and should shout out and identify the color on each ball as soon as possible after the ball leaves the pitcher's hand. This progression disciplines the athlete and increases the success rate of hitting the regulation-size ball later. The key to improving eye–hand coordination is to locate and identify the ball as early as possible.

Competition

Count the number of balls hit out of 20. Tipped balls count as hits. Assign 1 point for a tipped or foul ball, 2 points if the tipped ball is correctly identified, 3 points for all solid contacts, or 4 points for solid contact and correct identification. Record the total number of points for every 20 pitches; the maximum number of points that can be scored is 80. Athletes self-measure and track their personal best.

In Motion Hand–Eye Coordination

Age Range

8 to 14

Purpose

To improve eye–hand coordination by making contact with a moving object while on the move

Benefits

This skill is used primarily in tennis but is useful for athletes in general because it trains the eyes to track the ball while in motion and in various positions and situations. This skill helps develop catching skills for baseball, basketball, football, and lacrosse.

Equipment

One tennis racket per athlete, 20 tennis balls, four flat rubber dots

Setup

Create an area 15 yards by 15 yards on a hard surface, preferably a tennis court, but any hard service will do.

Execution

This drill focuses on hitting a ball while on the move. Three progressions advance and challenge athletes to focus on the ball in order to make consistent contact.

Progression 1

Place a rubber dot about 5 yards laterally from the athlete on each side. Begin with a partner continuously feeding tennis balls on one bounce, alternating to the right and left dots. The athlete hits the ball, which must pass a line 10 yards downcourt from the dots and stay within the width of the two dots. As soon as the athlete hits a ball, the next ball is served to the next dot until all 20 tennis balls have been served.

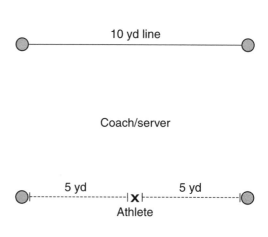

Competition

Record how many balls are hit after only one bounce and returned beyond the marked 10-yard line. Award 1 point for each ball hit after only one bounce and a second point for returning the ball between the two lateral dots. A maximum of 40 points can be scored.

Progression 2

Advance the drill by having the server toss balls to the two lateral dots without a bounce. The athlete must make contact prior to the ball bouncing and return the ball within the width of the two lateral dots marked 10 yards downcourt. The partner serves balls to each dot, alternating continuously without stopping. As soon as the athlete hits a ball, the next ball is served to the next dot until all 20 tennis balls have been served.

Competition

Record the number of successful returns beyond the marked line 10 yards downcourt within the width of the two dots. Award 1 point for each ball hit without a bounce and a second point for returning the ball between the two dots 10 yards downcourt. A maximum of 40 points can be scored.

Progression 3

Advance the drill by asking athletes to stand with their backs to the server. Once the server releases the ball to a specific dot, he or she yells for the athlete to turn. The athlete must find the ball, get to it, and hit it across the line 10 yards downcourt. Repeat the drill 10 times with a bounce and then 10 times without a bounce.

Competition

Record the number of balls successfully returned 10 yards downcourt within the boundaries of the two dots. Award 1 point for each ball hit after only one bounce and another point for returning the ball between the two dots downcourt for a maximum of 20 points.

Award 2 points for each ball hit with no bounces and 4 points for each ball hit with no bounce and successfully returned between the two dots downcourt for a maximum of 40 points.

Football Coordination

Age Range

8 to 14

Purpose

To improve eye–hand coordination and overall body coordination and awareness for football players

Equipment

You'll need a football (junior size for 8- to 12-year-olds, intermediate size for 13- and 14-year-olds), four cones, two 6-inch hurdles, and some chalk.

Setup

Square off an area 15 × 15 yards using four cones. Line one side with a six- to eight-foot chalk line (or use an athletic field with lines already marked).

Execution

The four progressions begin with athletes executing sideline catches while controlling the feet inbounds (one and two feet); this is followed by one-handed sideline catches and then behind-the-back catches.

Progression 1

The first progression involves throwing passes traveling out of bounds to the athlete on the sidelines, making him or her stretch out to catch the ball. Athletes must first attempt to keep two feet inbounds while catching the ball and then to keep one foot inbounds. The objective is to train the body to simultaneously coordinate two tasks (catching a ball and controlling the feet). Reverse direction after every 10 sets of throws and catches in order to replicate receiving a pass along the opposite side of the field. Once athletes are comfortable making catches along the sideline, advance to the second progression.

Progression 2

Advance the drill by placing a six-inch hurdle along the sideline and asking athletes to run toward the hurdle, leap over it with two feet at the same time, and immediately stretch to catch a ball traveling out of bounds. Reverse direction after every 10 throws. Repeat the drill, but have each athlete leap over the hurdle while attempting to stretch to catch a ball traveling out of bounds and to land with one foot inbounds. Reverse direction after 10 throws.

Competition

Attempt 10 consecutive catches and award 1 point for each successful catch made after jumping over the six-inch hurdle and landing with both feet inbounds while outstretched over the sideline. Follow this by attempting 10 consecutive catches and awarding 2 points for each successful catch made after jumping over the six-inch hurdle and landing with one foot inbounds while outstretched over the sideline. A maximum of 30 points can be scored.

Progression 3

Continue to throw passes traveling out of bounds to the athlete on the sideline, but advance the drill by challenging the athlete to make one-handed catches while stretched out over the sideline with both feet inbounds. Follow this with catches while keeping only one foot inbounds.

Competition

Attempt 10 consecutive catches, awarding 2 points for each successful one-handed catch made landing with both feet inbounds while outstretched over the sideline. Follow by attempting 10 consecutive catches and awarding 4 points for each successful catch made landing with one foot inbounds while outstretched over the sideline. A maximum of 60 points can be scored.

Progression 4

Advance the drill to include each athlete attempting to make behind-the-back catches along the sideline while keeping one or two feet inbounds. The objectives are to learn total body control and to maintain focus while executing multiple tasks with a raised degree of difficulty. This drill should be attempted only after athletes have success with one-handed catches along the sideline. Don't try this progression with athletes under the age of 13.

Competition

Attempt 10 consecutive catches and award 10 points for each successful behind-the-back catch made along the sideline. A maximum of 100 points can be scored.

Lacrosse Coordination

Age Range

8 to 14

Purpose

To improve eye–hand coordination while introducing a sight obstruction to the drill to help improve focus and overall body awareness

Benefits

Overall body awareness, eye–hand coordination, and sharp focus are
essential to executing many of the basic skills in the fast-paced game
of lacrosse.

Equipment

Four lacrosse balls, one lacrosse net, two lacrosse sticks, one football
goalpost

Setup

Place a lacrosse goal 10 feet directly behind a football goalpost. Athletes
stand about 10 feet on the other side of the football goalpost opposite
the lacrosse goal. A partner or coach stands on the lacrosse-goal side
of the football goalpost with four lacrosse balls.

Execution

Two progressions begin with
athletes running side to side
(marked by two cones six yards
apart) about 10 feet in front of
the football goalpost (which
acts as an obstruction to block
the athlete's view). This drill
attempts to replicate a gamelike
situation in which the athlete's
line of sight is obstructed as he
or she tries to catch, pass, and
shoot balls.

Net

10 ft

X Coach

10 ft

6 yd

Progression 1

The coach or playing partner
serves a total of 10 lacrosse balls
to the athlete unannounced as he or she passes in front of the football
goalpost (left to right and right to left), equally changing up the side

the ball is served to. At any moment, the athlete must successfully catch the ball on one side of the football goalpost and immediately laterally return to the other side of the post to shoot on goal.

Competition

Athletes attempt a total of 10 catches per competition. Award 1 point for each successful catch and 1 point for each successful shot that scores on goal. Be sure to equally distribute the passes to each side of the football goalpost, and make sure the shot is taken on goal as soon as the athlete passes the football goalpost. A maximum of 20 points can be scored.

Progression 2

A coach or playing partner serves lacrosse balls to athletes unannounced as they pass in front of the football goalpost (left to right and right to left), equally changing up the side to which the ball is served. Similar to progression 1, the athlete at any moment must successfully catch a ball on one side of the football goalpost as he or she passes from left to right and right to left and then immediately execute a 180-degree pivot and return to the other side of the post to shoot on goal.

Competition

Athletes attempt 10 catches per competition. Award 1 point for each successful catch and 180-degree pivot and return to the opposite side. Award 2 more points for each successful shot scored on goal. Be sure to equally distribute the passes to each side of the football goalpost, and make sure the shot is taken on goal as soon as the athlete passes the football goalpost. A maximum of 30 points can be scored.

CHAPTER 5

Build Balance

Proper balance involves a particular state of equilibrium or equipoise. The human balance system works with the visual and skeletal systems (the muscles and joints and their sensors) to maintain orientation. The three sensory systems used to maintain orientation, or balance, are the eyes, the inner ear, and nerve endings found in muscles, tendons, and joints that provide a sense of the body's position when placed in different situations. For example, when you're skiing, visual signals regarding your body's position begin at the brain, where sensory signals travel throughout your body, including sensors located on the bottom of your feet. These signals allow you to find and maintain balance in relation to your surroundings. To develop balance, you need to develop "muscle memory" (as discussed in chapter 4), an unconscious tensing and releasing of the right muscles in just the right increments that enables them to maintain their equilibrium in motion. It is through this process, for example, that a person learns to ride a bike. When learning, the body sends signals to the brain to orient the body to where it should be positioned and maintained, allowing the body's muscle memory to eventually take over and become what seems to be second nature.

Balance is the most essential skill for an athlete to possess, and time needs to be spent on developing it. All sports rely heavily on balance. Think of a soccer player attempting to keep possession of a ball, a pitcher winding up and throwing to home plate, a basketball player taking a jump shot, a football lineman blocking a defender, or a tennis player playing serve and volley. In each case, balance plays a key role in achieving the precise set of movements necessary for the skill to be performed correctly.

Without balance we would have no rhythm or fluidity to execute and coordinate the movement of body parts while maintaining the stable position required to perform the multiple tasks. Watch a highly skilled NBA player dribble, move, and glide through the air toward the basket, or an NHL player move up the ice with the puck and quickly transition into taking a shot, or a PGA player's golf swing—they all possess the same qualities. Four of the seven athletic components (agility, coordination, speed, and strength) rely on balance to be performed effectively.

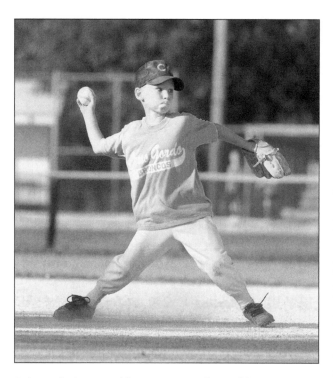

Balance helps an athlete maintain the stable position required for performing sport-specific tasks, such as throwing a baseball.

For example, the coordination of an effective baseball, golf, or tennis swing would not be possible without proper balance.

A key element in athletics is the ability to maintain balance while in motion. Whether you are rapidly transferring body weight during a golf swing, swinging or hitting and getting out of the batter's box in baseball, snowboarding down a mountain, or maneuvering around an opponent in ice hockey, soccer, or lacrosse, balance plays a primary role in the execution of most athletic movements. Balance allows the body to transfer weight while performing. Athletes need to be able to continue to execute while transitioning from a variety of body positions and movements. They often find themselves off balance before or after executing a play. To be in a position to finish a play, or to prepare for the next play, they must be able to adjust quickly to regain proper balance.

Balance develops an overall sense of equilibrium, self-control, and total body awareness. We consider balance the foundation to athletic development. The more balance becomes the focus of a child's athletic development, the more adept he or she will become at performing more difficult and complicated tasks, such as turning a double-play in baseball, throwing a football on a full run, changing body direction in midair to avoid a defender when driving to the basket, skating and stick-handling the length of the ice while avoiding defenders, and so on.

This chapter contains drills and competitions that develop a child's balance and help create a greater sense of how to control the body in many athletic situations. We include drills to develop balance from a static position, while in motion, and with or without a partner. We want to provide your athletes with the proper foundation to succeed in sports, as well as an essential health benefit for years to come. Balance training improves the core strength and stability of the body and is a prevention measure for future back and hip injuries that plague many of us in adulthood. Balance training should become a focus.

Balance in Motion

Age Range

8 to 14

Purpose

To increase overall balance and aid in recovering from off-balanced positions

Benefits

Athletes develop equilibrium in motion through muscle memory. Balance is essential to all sports that require movement and is the foundation on which other athletic components are built.

Equipment

A wooden two-by-four about 8 to 10 feet long, two tennis balls, one 6-inch and one 12-inch high hurdle

Setup

Place the two-by-four flat on the ground. Athletes execute the drill by moving the full length and back each rotation.

Execution

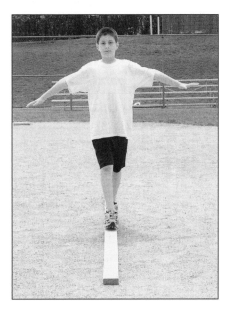

There are seven progressions that help athletes develop a sense of equilibrium when in motion. The progressions slowly advance to include athletes performing multiple tasks and movement as they develop equilibrium. For safety purposes, we recommend a spotter to walk the length of the two-by-four as kids perform the tasks.

Progression 1

Athletes walk the length of the two-by-four beam four times, attempting not to lose balance and step off. Once they reach the other end, they immediately return to the starting point, this time walking backward. Allow athletes to look at their feet and look behind them for the first time through, but after that, tell them to look up and straight ahead for the remainder of the routine.

Progression 2

Athletes repeat the forward and backward walk on the beam four times but add a 180-degree rotation for a forward approach and a 360-degree rotation for a backward approach when they finish at each end of the beam. This can be accomplished by lifting up onto the balls of the feet and rotating with the hips, without lifting the feet off the beam, and extending both arms out to the sides. As kids become more comfortable, they might find they no longer need to extend their arms to maintain balance. They continue to walk either backward or forward across the beam.

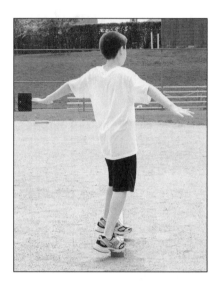

Progression 3

Athletes walk forward and backward across the beam four times as in progression 1, but now they try to catch tennis balls thrown to them from 10 feet away. Each athlete should try to reach and catch the ball while maintaining balance on the beam. Balls should be tossed from a variety of directions, both in front of the athletes and behind them and both low and high.

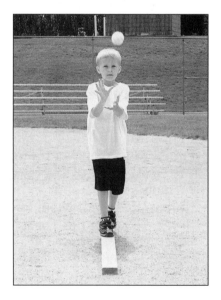

 Competition

Athletes catch and return tennis balls by tossing as many balls as they can over 60 seconds back and forth to a partner. They must continue to move on the beam for each catch to count. Record the number of successful catches made without falling off the beam, awarding 1 point for each ball caught and another point for each ball accurately tossed to the partner. If an athlete falls off the beam, the count starts over from zero.

Progression 4

The athlete walks across the wooden beam as in progression 1. This time each athlete should toss two tennis balls up in the air and then catch them. The balls are tossed straight up in the air to the same hand simultaneously; there is no transfer of balls from hand to hand.

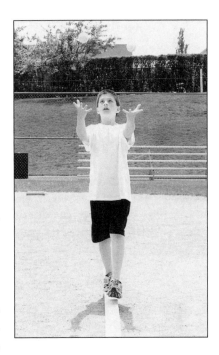

Progression 5

Athletes pick up the pace of the walk forward and backward on the beam without falling off.

Progression 6

Each athlete walks laterally (sideways) by crossing one foot over the other (a), stepping to the side with the other foot (b), and then crossing the first foot behind the other foot. Athletes cross the beam and return to the other end facing the same direction. After perfecting this without stepping off the beam, they increase speed.

To further progress each stage of this drill, have athletes step over one 6-inch hurdle and one 12-inch hurdle placed on the ground over the two-by-four beam. As a safety precaution, have a spotter reverse hurdles in the correct direction each time an athlete passes over a hurdle.

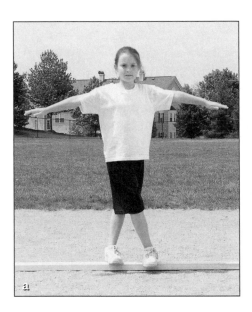

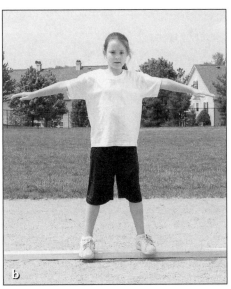

Record how long it takes athletes to execute six passes across the beam (a pass equals one time across the length of the beam); add three seconds for each fall off the beam.

Progression 7

This progression adds a partner to the drill. Place two 8- to 10-foot two-by-fours flat on the ground next to each other (touching) width-wise. Athletes start from opposite ends and walk toward each other and pass without touching or stopping. After they can do this, they perform the six previous progressions but this time with a partner. To increase difficulty, use one two-by-four instead of two. Repeat until each athlete begins to successfully execute the drill on a consistent basis.

DRILL 5.2
Knee Balancing

Age Range

8 to 14

Purpose

To increase overall balance in various situations; to aid in recovering from off-balanced positions

Benefits

Athletes develop equilibrium in motion through muscle memory. To develop balance, athletes must develop muscle memory in the core of their bodies (abdomen, lower back, and hips).

Equipment

You'll need a Vew-Do zone balance board or a half foam roll. A Vew-Do zone balance board is a flat, wooden, oval-shaped board with three fulcrum attachments on the bottom to increase difficulty in maintaining balance. You can find Vew-Do zone balance boards at sporting goods stores or at www.Vewdo.com.

Setup

Place the Vew-Do boards or half rolls on a semihard carpet or hard gymnastics mat.

Execution

There are two progressions for this drill.

Progression 1

Each athlete starts on hands and knees with both knees placed on the board or roll. Ask the athlete to lift one foot off the ground while maintaining balance with both hands placed on the board to each side of the knees *(a)*; the other foot should be placed on the ground with only the tips of the toes touching. The first foot is lifted several inches off the ground, and the knee remains bent slightly. Over time, each athlete works toward fully extending the leg back and locking the knee while making the back parallel to the ground *(b)*. Alternate lifting each foot off the ground while maintaining balance, and then attempt to lift both feet off the ground simultaneously, keeping knees bent and hands placed on the board (or roll) on each side of the knees.

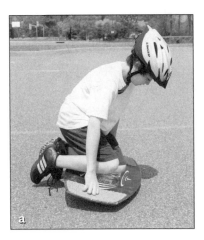 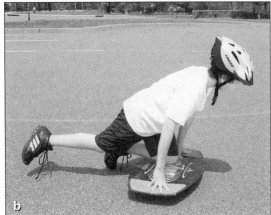

Progression 2

The athletes lift both hands off their boards (or rolls) and both feet off the ground while maintaining balance as long as they can on their knees. They might find that lifting both arms up and out to the sides allows them to gain and maintain their balance faster and longer.

🎗 Competition

Record how long each athlete can remain balanced before falling off the balance board or half

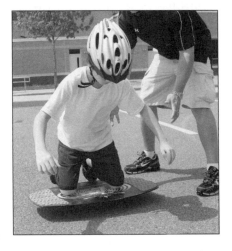

foam roll. Record each athlete's total time spent balancing over five attempts. For a total competition score, award 1 point for each second that an athlete maintains balance on the board (or roll) for all five attempts combined.

Balance Boarding

Age Range

8 to 14

Purpose

To increase overall balance in various situations; to aid in recovering from off-balanced positions while executing sport fundamentals such as catching and throwing

Benefits

Athletes develop equilibrium in motion through muscle memory. To develop balance, athletes must develop muscle memory in the sensory nerves through their lower limbs and bottoms of their feet.

Equipment

A Vew-Do zone balance board or half foam roll

Setup

Place the Vew-Do boards or half rolls on a semihard carpet or hard gymnastics mat. Be sure to use spotters to prevent athletes from falling and hurting themselves. Athletes should also wear protective helmets during this drill and the competitions.

Execution

There are two progressions. The drill begins with a simple balance technique and is followed by adding specific sport functions.

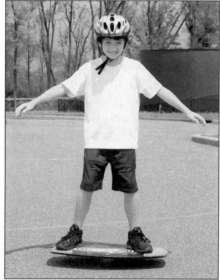

Progression 1

Start the drill by placing the teeter fulcrum on the bottom of the Vew-Do zone board. If you don't have access to a Vew-Do board, use a half foam roll (found in the fitness section of most sporting goods stores). Athletes attempt to maintain balance on the board while standing. Over time, once athletes become accustomed to balancing themselves, advance to the competition phase of the drill.

Competition

Record each athlete's total amount of time spent balancing on the board over five attempts. For a total competition score, award 1 point for each second that an athlete maintains balance on the board (or roll) during all five attempts.

Progression 2

Introduce athletes to balancing while focusing on executing other athletic skills simultaneously. An athlete stands on the board, as in progression 1, and tosses a basketball, football, or tennis ball to a partner. The partner catches the ball and tosses it back while balancing on a board. A variation of this drill for athletes 12 years old and older is to throw them light medicine balls. This further tests their overall balance by having them react and adjust to the added weight while focusing on executing the catch and throw.

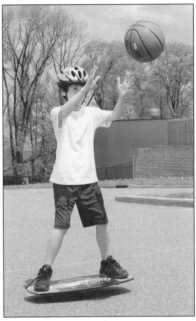

Competition

Record for each athlete the total amount of time balanced and total number of successful catches over five combined attempts. Award 1 point for each second that an athlete maintains balance on the board (or roll) and another point for each successful catch. Combine all five attempts for a total competition score.

DRILL 5.4
Balancing in Different Body Positions

Age Range

8 to 14

Purpose

To increase overall balance when placed in different body positions

Benefits

Athletes develop equilibrium in motion through muscle memory. In hockey, football, soccer, basketball, or lacrosse competition, athletes often find themselves in awkward positions in which they need to maintain balance to continue with play. A running back in football, for example, might be hit and spun around, nearly hitting the ground, requiring a keen sense of balance to stay on his feet and continue running downfield.

Equipment

A Vew-Do zone balance board or half foam roll

Setup

Place the Vew-Do boards or half rolls on a semihard carpet or hard gymnastics mat. Be sure spotters are available at all times to prevent athletes from falling. Protective helmets are recommended for this drill.

Execution

This drill can be extremely difficult and should be introduced only after athletes can successfully execute the previous balance boarding drill. The athlete begins by squatting on the balance board with the left hand touching the lower part of the right leg. The body twists to the right, and the right arm is either used for balance or positioned behind the back for more of a challenge. The athlete executes the drill in different directions, switching hands and touching the opposite leg.

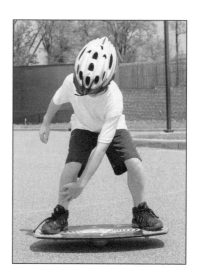

Competition

Record each athlete's total time spent balancing over a total of five attempts. For a total competition score, award 1 point for each second that an athlete maintains balance on the board (or roll) for all five attempts combined.

DRILL 5.5

Bicycle Balance

Age Range

8 to 14

Purpose

To increase overall balance by using a nontraditional training tool—the bicycle

Benefits

One of the main skills kids master at a young age is balancing on a bicycle. Bike riding can also be used to continue to increase an athlete's overall balance skills and to develop the body's equilibrium in motion through muscle memory. A key element to accelerating a child's learning experience is to engage him or her in a variety of enjoyable activities. Most children know how to ride a bike, but they have likely never used their bikes as tools to enhance their athletic skills within an organized practice. You might also consider having your athletes bring their bicycles to an organized baseball, basketball, football, soccer, or lacrosse practice.

Equipment

A mountain bike or BMX bike and a protective bike helmet

Setup

You can conduct these drills in your driveway or an empty parking lot, on grass, or on a dirt path. Use spotters to prevent athletes from falling. Spotters should run alongside athletes when the bike is moving and catch athletes if they fall. All bicyclists should wear protective bike helmets.

Execution

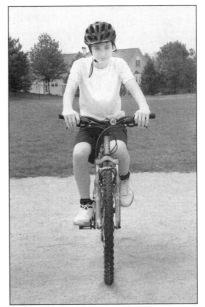

There are seven progressions that advance from simple balancing to complex variations.

Progression 1

Each athlete sits on the seat of the bike with both feet on the pedals. Hands are on each side of the handlebars. Remind them to focus the center of the bike equally between the two legs at all times with arms steady on the handlebars.

🏅 **Competition**

Record how long they can keep their bikes balanced without placing their feet on the ground. Use a point system similar to the other competitions, awarding 1 point for each second the bike is held balanced and the athlete's feet have not touched the ground. Each athlete's progress is measured by the increase in time spent balanced on the bike. Record a personal-best score for five total attempts, and add that score to the personal-best scores of the remaining six competitions executed for this drill.

Progression 2

Have each athlete stand on both pedals with hands placed on the handlebars to stabilize the bike. If they struggle with this, have them focus on keeping the bike centered an equal distance between the two legs.

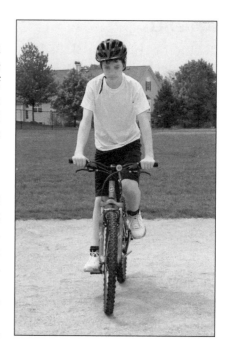

🏅 **Competition**

Record how long each athlete can stand on both pedals without placing a foot on the ground. Award 2 points for each second the bike is held balanced and the athlete's feet have not touched the ground. Record a personal-best score for five attempts, and add that score to the personal-best scores of all the other competitions for this drill.

Progression 3

Each athlete sits on the seat of the bike with both feet on the pedals and one hand off the handlebars.

🏅 **Competition**

Record how long each athlete can keep the bike balanced on the two tires without placing the feet on the ground. Award 3 points for each second the bike is held balanced without feet touching the ground. Record a personal-best score for five attempts, and add that score to the personal-best scores of all the other competitions for this drill.

Progression 4

Each athlete sits on the seat of the bike with feet on the pedals and hands off the handlebars.

🏅 **Competition**

Record how long each athlete can keep the bike balanced on the two tires without placing the feet on the ground. Award 4 points for each second the bike is held balanced without feet touching the ground. Record a personal-best score for five attempts, and add that score to the personal-best scores of all the other competitions for this drill.

Progression 5

Have each athlete stand on one side of the bike on one pedal while holding onto the bike with two hands. Remind them to try to keep the tires straight by steadying the bike with two hands on the handlebars and the body slightly bent over the center of the bike. Once they can do this, have each athlete stand on one side of the bike on one pedal while holding onto the bike with only one hand. These techniques are difficult and should be carefully spotted.

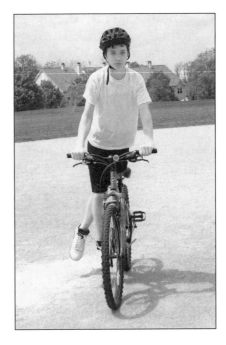

 Competition

Record how long each athlete can keep the bike balanced on the two tires without placing the feet on the ground. Award 5 points for each second the bike is held balanced without feet touching the ground. Record a personal-best score for five attempts, and add that score to the personal-best scores of all the other competitions for this drill.

Progression 6

The previous drills have been done in a stationary position, and now it's time to progress to using movement. Athletes ride their bikes a set distance (about 20 yards) at a moderate speed before applying both the front and back brakes equally and gliding to a complete stop. This is followed immediately by balancing the bike with both feet on the pedals and hands on the handlebars without placing either foot on the ground.

 Competition

Record how long each athlete can keep balanced on the bike before placing a foot on the ground. Award 6 points for each second the bike is held balanced without feet touching the ground. Record a personal-best score for five attempts, and add that score to the personal-best scores of all the other competitions for this drill.

Progression 7

Once athletes have consistent success in executing progression 6, have them repeat the 20-yard ride and stop. This time ask each athlete to swing one leg across the bike as it's moving and to place the foot on the same pedal as the other foot; tell the athletes to glide to a stop without applying the brakes. Speed and distance are not important factors in this drill. The focus is on the execution of swinging the leg over the bike and keeping the bike balanced after it stops.

🎗 Competition

Record how long each athlete can keep balanced after stopping and balancing on one pedal. Award 7 points for each second the bike is held balanced without feet touching the ground. Record a personal-best score for five attempts, and add that score to the personal-best scores of all the other competitions for this drill.

DRILL 5.6
Roll, Balance, and Run

Age Range

8 to 14

Purpose

To incorporate balance in different body positions; to maintain or regain balance after specific athletic movements

Benefits

This drill helps athletes develop equilibrium in motion through muscle memory. They improve in their ability to fall down, get back on their feet immediately, regain balance, and continue play.

Equipment

A tumbling mat (optional if on grass or turf), a poly balance beam 8 feet long by 4 inches wide by 1.5 inches thick

Setup

Place the balance beam on a semihard carpet or grass area at the end of a gymnastics tumbling mat. If the beam tends to move when athletes land on it, have someone hold the far end down with a foot. If a mat is unavailable, a soft carpet or grass area works fine.

Execution

Two progressions are designed for advanced athletes who have mastered the other balance drills in the chapter.

Progression 1

An athlete stands about four feet from the balance beam and executes a forward roll *(a, b)*. The athlete tries to place both feet on the balance beam near the end of the forward roll *(c)* and finishes in a standing position on the beam *(d)*. She then immediately moves forward to the end of the beam without losing balance.

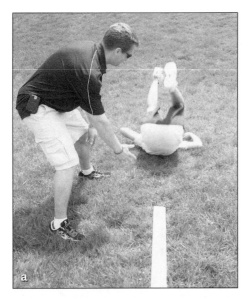

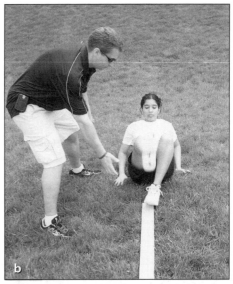

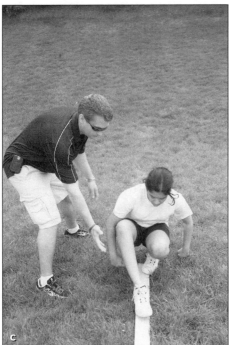

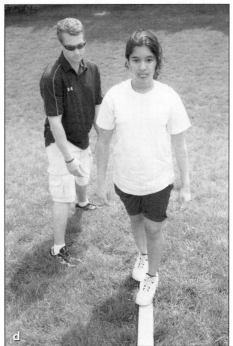

Progression 2

Progress the drill by moving athletes back and having them slowly approach the mat by walking into one forward roll immediately onto the balance beam and finishing with a run to the end of the beam. A spotter follows athletes into the forward roll to watch and protect their necks. A spotter is also near the balance beam, prepared to catch athletes if they begin to fall.

Tennis Balancing

Age Range

8 to 14

Purpose

To get better at executing tennis shots while unstable and off balance

Benefits

Athletes develop equilibrium in motion through muscle memory. Tennis players often find themselves in awkward positions when trying to reach balls or hit shots. This drill forces athletes to execute in uncomfortable or unstable positions.

Equipment

Four half foam rolls, 12 tennis balls, a tennis racket

Setup

Place the four rolls in the center of one half of a tennis court on the middle and top of the two service boxes about two feet from the top of the service box toward the net.

Execution

A partner or feeder bounces balls to each side of the athlete. Have the athlete walk forward and backward on the half foam rolls while hitting balls over the net inbounds for two minutes.

Competition

Award 1 point for every ball struck and 1 point for every ball hit inbounds prior to stepping off the half foam rolls. If an athlete falls off the foam rolls, record the points scored and repeat; record until two minutes have elapsed.

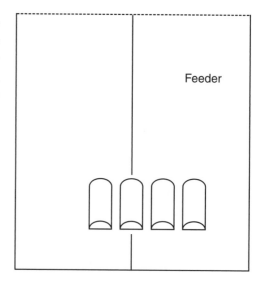

Feeder

Basketball Balancing

Age Range

8 to 14

Purpose

To execute basketball shots while off balance and unstable

Benefits

Athletes develop equilibrium in motion through muscle memory. Basketball players often find themselves in awkward positions when trying to get shots off. This drill places athletes in uncomfortable or unstable positions while executing shots.

Equipment

Vew-Do zone balance board, three basketballs

Setup

Place the Vew-Do board in front of a basket. A partner is positioned under the basket to feed basketballs to the athlete.

Execution

The athlete begins by balancing on the balance board. The partner then begins feeding basketballs in the air for the athlete to catch and shoot for two minutes. Feeding balls on one bounce to the athlete can adjust the drill.

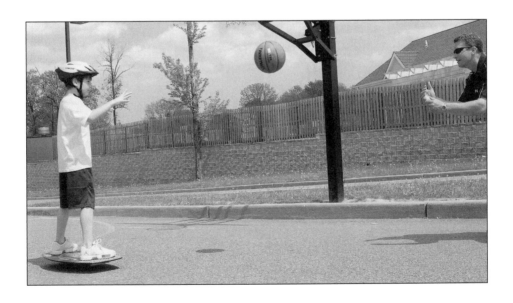

Competition

Award 1 point for every ball caught and 2 points for every basket made prior to falling off the balance board. Each competition runs a total of two minutes. Record the most points recorded prior to falling off the board.

CHAPTER 6

Boost Stamina

Stamina is what gives athletes enduring physical or mental energy and strength and allows them to keep going over an extended period of time. Although stamina is typically associated with endurance athletes such as marathon runners, triathletes, and cyclists, every sport or athletic activity involves stamina. The obvious sports that require a focus on stamina include soccer, lacrosse, ice hockey, basketball, football, and tennis. Each of these sports involves continuous play with no regular rest intervals such as those that occur between pitches and innings in baseball, for example. Sports such as baseball and softball are slow paced with little extended physical exertion, unless you're a pitcher or catcher. Still, baseball is a sport in which stamina must be developed in order to develop strength (which we'll discuss in chapter 7). All sports have specific stamina requirements that need to be developed for athletes to perform at optimal levels.

Stamina allows athletes to execute the skills of their sport without tiring or losing concentration. When athletes find themselves tiring during a competition, they might become physically unable to execute the skills necessary to excel. For example, a hockey defenseman who tires toward the end of a game might be unable to chase down a puck in his own zone, allowing the opposition to gain control and score. Fatigue can also affect concentration and decision making, such as when a basketball point guard gets tired and misses a pick set by a teammate and ends up turning the ball over at a critical point in the game.

Today's kids spend a great deal of time in front of computers, video games, and television sets. They are sedentary for long periods of time at school, including the commute to and from school, with little to no movement other than walking between classes and to lunch. The reduction and, in some cases, elimination of physical education has drastically decreased physical activity during school hours. In addition, more school systems are finding it difficult to continue after-school activities and sports because of budget restraints. These factors combined have led to a serious decline in overall fitness among a majority of kids and can be quite noticeable when a child plays on an organized sports team.

Kids still enjoy running and moving and the freedom that play provides. But for many, the only chance they have to exercise their stamina is at an organized practice or game. In these settings, endurance does not receive enough attention or is presented in a negative fashion. Unfortunately, stamina training is often applied as a punishment. Athletes are sent to run a number of laps or told to do a number of push-ups as a punishment for being late, making a mistake, or misbehaving. This can result in a lifetime of negative feelings toward working out. Because endurance is such an integral part of sport performance, stamina training should never be used as a punishment. It should be presented as a fun activity that promotes positive feelings toward working out.

Stamina training should be done strategically. It should not necessarily be conducted in its entirety at one particular time during a practice. Splitting up stamina training within a practice should increase the overall intensity each athlete exerts during these segments. For best results, stamina training should be customized depending on age and placed appropriately within a practice. We approach stamina training in two different phases: general physical conditioning (primarily for ages 8 through 14) and sport-specific training (for ages 10 through 14). For our purposes here we'll focus on general physical conditioning and touch only briefly on sport-specific training. Stamina is important when training for any sport. Sport-specific conditioning is not absolutely necessary for kids at this age as long as they're getting general conditioning. You can be creative in your approach to general stamina training when conditioning sport-specific athletes to help them receive optimal benefits.

Stamina training for kids should consist of general activities that are fun and that encourage the athletes to push themselves to their next

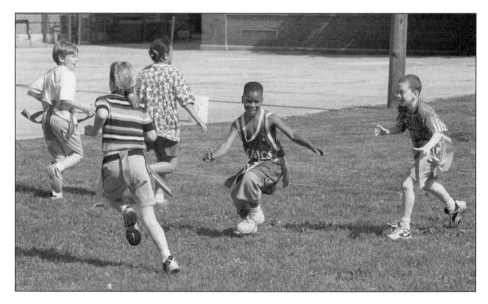

To promote positive attitudes toward working out and to keep kids interested in the task at hand, stamina training should be structured as fun and enjoyable activities.

level of fitness. Many healthy kids of this age have a natural supply of energy that provides them with significant endurance to apply to any athletic event they wish. But because of the sedentary nature of American society today, stamina training should not be overlooked.

One of the best general methods for conditioning stamina in young kids is to incorporate different sports into your practices. For example, if you coach basketball, take six to nine minutes twice a practice to play small-sided games of soccer, lacrosse, or flag football. This allows your athletes to perform movements not associated with their sport and is an excellent way to quickly improve overall stamina. Plus the games make practice more fresh and fun. Playing a game of ultimate Frisbee is another option. Ultimate Frisbee is played on college campuses as a recreational activity and is a great conditioning activity that provides plenty of fun competition and distracts the athlete's attention away from fatigue. See pages 93 to 94 for a description of ultimate Frisbee.

Another option is obstacle courses, which can be the most effective way to execute a training routine in a fun and creative way. Very few athletes truly enjoy stamina training, but nearly everyone enjoys the variety and challenge of an obstacle course. This is a way to involve athletes in stamina training while having them execute and focus on other athletic elements, such as coordination, speed, and strength, as they begin to become fatigued.

When possible, set up your obstacle courses on diverse terrains. There are two reasons for this: to avoid boring your athletes by giving them fresh challenges, and because if the body repeats the same routine over and over, it begins to adjust and master those particular movements, which reduces the conditioning effect. You might place part of the course on the side of a hill that athletes must climb while performing a routine such as a slalom around cones. If you have access to a beach or sand, you can introduce digging or climbing out of holes into your course. (Note that sand increases the overall intensity of a workout, so your course should be shorter.) Or you can take your team to a running trail; many communities have developed trails with multiple manmade fitness stations. If trails don't have fitness stations, develop your own natural ones, such as pull-ups on secure tree branches, push-ups off logs, and so on. When developing obstacle courses, be sure to change them regularly to give athletes new challenges and to work on different body movements, which accelerates their overall fitness progression. See pages 84 to 88 for sample obstacle courses.

One obvious method of stamina training, and the most common, is running. Endurance training for most sports is associated with doing laps around a field or track, and with good reason—when combined with other forms of stamina training, running is a great way to build athletic endurance. And if presented correctly, running can be fun. If you're on a track, it's a good idea to vary the type of running you have your athletes do. This is because most athletes don't run at one constant speed in their sport; most sports require athletes to execute sprints, jogs, instant accelerations, sudden slow-downs, and rapid changes of direction. A mix of speeds and types of running also allows your athletes to work different muscle groups. For an example of incorporating different forms of running into a track workout, see pages 88 to 89.

In general, endurance training on a track should be reserved for athletes 10 and older because these kids are more focused and not as apt to become bored with training of this nature. Younger kids should stick to activity-based training that's game oriented and that serves to misdirect their attention from a focus on running.

You might consider taking your athletes running at nontraditional locations, such as a swimming pool. The resistance athletes receive when running through water builds overall stamina while avoiding the wear and tear of running on dry ground. Pool-running is often conducted in the deep end of a swimming pool under close supervision of an adult who can swim and is trained in water safety. Athletes should tread water by using their normal running stride, as if they were running on a track. Until athletes perfect this drill, are comfortable in the water, and can swim, they should wear lifejackets or flotation belts. See page 93 for a pool-running workout.

DRILL 6.1
▰▰▰ Stamina Course for Younger Kids ▰▰▰

Age Range

8 to 9

Purpose

To prepare an athlete's overall stamina for numerous activities and competitions

Benefits

Athletes build the stamina they need to execute skills effectively when they become fatigued over the course of competition.

Equipment

30 cones, two 3-pound fitness balls, 24 low track hurdles, two 10-pound medicine balls, 20 12-inch hurdles, a stopwatch, a whistle

Setup

Six athletes participate simultaneously while others work at other drills. Athletes rotate into this drill every six minutes. Set up a 50-yard by 30-yard area on a football field or other grassy area. Set up three 10-yard lanes adjacent to each other and outlined by 10 cones; one lane is 50 yards long, the second is 30 yards long, and the third is 20 yards long. Assign two athletes to each lane. Rotate each lane every two minutes until all three lanes have been completed, for a total of six minutes.

Each lane requires different tasks to be conducted for two minutes each. The 50-yard lane is set up with two adjacent slalom courses (marked by 20 cones in two separate rows, arranged in a zigzag formation five yards apart downfield and five yards to each alternating side; see diagram). Place two 3-pound fitness balls at the starting line of this lane. The 30-yard lane is set up with two adjacent lines of 10 consecutive 12-inch hurdles, arranged 1 yard apart for a total of 10 yards, beginning 10 yards from the starting line and 10 yards from the end of the lane. Adjacent to the 12-inch hurdles, place two adjacent rows of 12 low track hurdles (adjust a track hurdle to it's lowest setting height), arranged 2 yards apart for a total of 24 yards (placed 3 yards from each end of the 30-yard lane). The third 20-yard lane is outlined simply by four cones; two 10-pound medicine balls are placed at the starting line of the lane.

Execution

Begin with two athletes assigned to each lane. Every two minutes blow a whistle and rotate each group of two athletes to their next assigned lane until all three lanes have been completed. Count the total number of completed up-and-back executions of the tasks assigned to each lane over the two minutes.

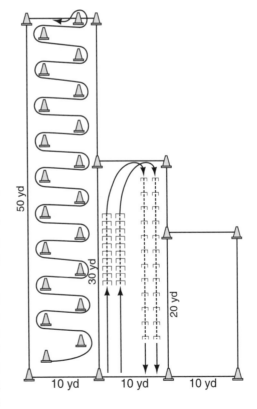

- The 50-yard lane's task is running the slalom up and back, followed immediately by carrying a three-pound fitness ball on the same slalom course up and back.

- The 30-yard lane consists of jumping over the 10 consecutive 12-inch hurdles up the lane, followed immediately by alternating over and under each of the 12 consecutive low track hurdles back down the lane to the original starting line.

- The 20-yard lane requires the athlete to travel on all fours (hands and feet) up and down the lane, followed immediately by rolling a 10-pound medicine ball up and back.

🏅 Competition

For a total of six consecutive minutes, count the total number of passes made for each lane and award 2 points for each pass on the 50-yard lane, 6 points for each pass on the 30-yard lane, and 10 points for each pass on the 20-yard lane. Athletes can self-measure their progress by adding the total number of points they accumulate over each six-minute interval. Competitions can also pit teams or individual athletes against each other by totaling up accumulated scores.

DRILL 6.2
Stamina Course for Older Kids

Age Range

10 to 14

Purpose

To improve an athlete's stamina in the later stages of competition

Benefits

Athletes build the stamina they need to execute skills effectively toward the end of competitions or when they become fatigued over the course of competition.

Equipment

Four cones, two 12-pound medicine balls, six low track hurdles, 10 12-inch hurdles, a stopwatch, a whistle

Setup

Set up a circle 15 yards from the center point to each of four cones positioned equally around the perimeter on grass or turf. Two athletes participate at once in a circle while other athletes do other drills. Athletes rotate into this drill every three minutes.

Execution

Assign each athlete to a cone on opposite sides of the circle, 30 yards apart. Give each athlete a 12-pound medicine ball that is carried from one cone to the next after completing each task. Every task executed from each cone requires the athlete to travel in a straight line to the center point of the circle and back before rotating counterclockwise around the perimeter of the circle. After starting the drill, keep time on a stopwatch until three minutes have elapsed, and then blow a whistle to end the drill. Each cone requires different tasks to be completed.

The first station requires the athlete to run forward into the center of the circle, run backward toward the perimeter cone, and then repeat (note that this is the only station that is repeated before proceeding counterclockwise to the next station). The athlete then takes the assigned 12-pound medicine ball and runs counterclockwise to the next station. (This is repeated after the conclusion of each station.)

The second station requires the athlete to jump consecutively over 10 12-inch hurdles placed one yard apart, until reaching the center of the circle. The athlete then returns immediately by laterally jumping over each hurdle.

The third station involves traveling over and then under six low track hurdles both ways into and out of the circle.

The fourth station requires the athlete to crawl facedown on hands and feet into the center of the circle and then travel back face-up on the hands and feet.

This drill requires each athlete to complete as many laps as possible around the circle with the medicine ball in three minutes.

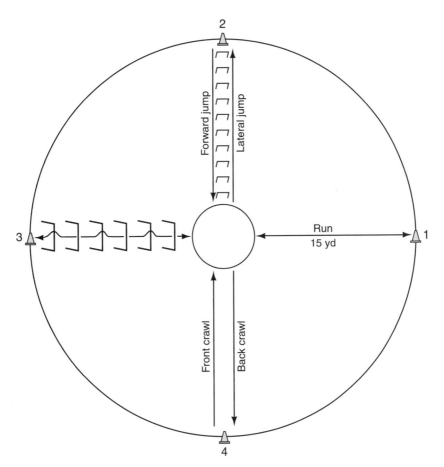

For three consecutive minutes count the number of laps completed around the circle. Award 5 points for each successfully completed lap. Athletes can self-measure their progress by adding the total number of points they accumulate over each three-minute interval. Competitions can also pit teams or individual athletes against each other by totaling up accumulated scores.

DRILL 6.3
Track Run

Age Range

10 to 14

Purpose

To build stamina with nontraditional drills

Benefits

Improves stamina by mixing up the typical training routine, keeping it fresh and challenging.

Equipment

Six cones, a stopwatch, a whistle

Setup

Six athletes prepare to run on a 400-meter running track. They start at the traditional starting line marked on the track.

Execution

Six athletes run counterclockwise around the running track. Assign one athlete per lane. Begin all athletes running at the same time in their assigned lanes. Alternate timed intervals in order of 30, 15, 10, 20, and 30 seconds, repeating the same timed intervals until you reach 4 minutes. The first 30-second interval is a straight run; the 15-second interval is a backward run; the 10-second interval is a run with high knees (athletes are on the balls of their feet lifting their knees as high as they can with each stride); the 20-second interval is a lateral run with hips squarely facing the inside of the track; and the final 30-second interval is a lateral run with hips squarely facing the outside of the track.

Athletes then repeat this sequence for four minutes, at which point they stop and mark on the track where they finished. Each athlete then immediately retrieves a cone at the center of the track and brings it to the finish point of the last interval. The athletes then begin running as fast as they can for another 60 seconds. At 60 seconds, blow the whistle and ask all athletes to freeze; then record the distance traveled by each athlete. This distance becomes their base by which to self-measure future performances.

Competition

Take the base distance recorded and award 1 point for each additional 20 meters covered over the five-minute drill; subtract 1 point for each 20 meters the athlete fails to complete before reaching their base distance. Note that each personal best becomes the athlete's new base by which he or she is measured in the future. Over the course of a season or consecutive training sessions, record each athlete's points and keep track to compare against earlier sessions and those of other athletes.

DRILL 6.4
Up and Down Track

Age Range

10 to 14

Purpose

To increase athletes' overall stamina and conditioning

Benefits

This conditioning drill works numerous parts of the body throughout the workout, training the body with a total-conditioning, rather than a one-dimensional, approach. Please note that this is an advanced stamina drill that can be difficult for athletes to master. We suggest introducing parts of this drill prior to running the drill in its entirety.

Equipment

A set of adjacent bleachers, twelve 12-inch hurdles, a two-foot high bench, a stopwatch, a whistle

Setup

Athletes prepare to run in the traditional counterclockwise direction around a 400-meter running track (or other measured-out perimeter). Start each athlete at the traditional starting line marked on the track. Start another athlete every 30 seconds.

Execution

Each athlete begins by running two 400-meter laps. On the third lap, athletes run up the bleachers stepping on every step to the top of the bleachers and back down. This is followed by running over 12 consecutive 12-inch hurdles at the 100-meter mark on the track. This is followed by 25 switches on a bench located at the 200-meter mark on the track (switches are executed by placing one leg up on the bench and exploding off that leg straight into the air while the athlete switches legs and lands on the opposite leg on the bench and immediately explodes straight up). They repeat the alternating switches a total of 25 times. Athletes then proceed another 100 meters until they reach a coned-off area, where they execute 25 push-ups. The fourth lap repeats the third-lap tasks with one difference at the first bleacher station. At

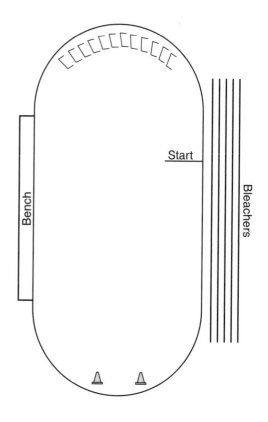

this station, the athlete ascends the bleachers hitting *every other* step before repeating all tasks from the third lap. The fifth lap repeats all tasks from the third and fourth laps except for the bleacher climb, in which the athlete ascends hitting every *third* step. The sixth and final lap is a 400-meter run with no additional tasks.

Competition

Record how long it takes to complete all six laps. Athletes should attempt to improve on their personal best each time they run the course.

DRILL 6.5
■ On- and Off-Track ■

Age Range

12 to 14

Purpose

To increase athletes' overall stamina

Benefits

Breaks up the monotony of track work by mixing up and introducing different conditioning challenges and movements. Please note that this is an advanced stamina drill that can be difficult for athletes to master. We suggest introducing parts of this drill prior to running the drill in its entirety.

Equipment

23 cones (11 orange cones and 12 yellow cones), a stopwatch, a whistle

Setup

This drill requires a 400-meter running track (or other measured-out perimeter) and a football or soccer field located in the middle of the track. Athletes prepare to run counterclockwise around the track. Each athlete starts at the starting line marked on the track. Start another athlete every 30 seconds. Place orange cones down the center of the football or soccer field at these positions: on the end line of one end zone, on the goal line of the same end zone, on the 25-yard line, on the 50-yard line, 75 yards out from the same end zone, and on the opposite goal line. Place yellow cones at these positions: on the goal line of the end zone, on the 10-yard line on the far sideline, on the 20-yard line at the center of the field, on the 30-yard line on the far sideline, on the 40-yard line at the center of the field, on the 50-yard line on the far sideline, at the center of the field on the 50-yard line, downfield on the 40-yard line near the sideline, on the 30-yard line at the center of the field, on the 20-yard line on the near sideline, on the 10-yard line at the center of the field, and on the goal line near the sideline. On an adjacent hill, place five cones five yards apart from right to left and five yards apart up the hill. If a hill is not available, place cones in a slalom course fashion on bleachers.

Execution

Athletes begin by running one 400-meter lap. They then move immediately (without resting) to the football field *(a)* inside the track area. They begin sprinting the 110-yard shuttle from the designated end of the field (at the back of the end zone) for 110 yards; jogging back upfield to the end-zone line and sprinting back downfield 100 yards; jogging back upfield to the 25-yard line and immediately sprinting back downfield 75 yards; jogging back to the 50-yard line and immediately sprinting downfield 50 yards; and returning back upfield 25 yards before sprinting back downfield 25 yards. Following this, they immediately begin running 400 meters around the track before running to the bottom of an adjacent hill and sprinting up and down a slalom course through the five cones placed on the hill a total of five times before returning to the track to complete another 400-meter lap. After completing the lap, they return immediately (without resting) to the football field's end zone and begin sprinting downfield on a slalom course, touching every designated yellow cone downfield *(b)*. They complete the drill by returning immediately to the track (without resting) to run a final 400-meter lap.

Competition

Record how long it takes each athlete to complete the course. Athletes self-measure and attempt to improve on their best time each time they run the course.

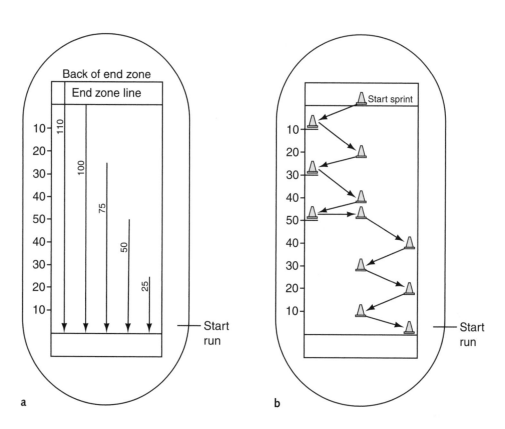

Water Running

Age Range

8 to 14

Purpose

To increase athletes' overall stamina

Benefits

Athletes build the stamina they need to execute skills effectively toward the end of competitions or when they become fatigued over the course of competition.

Equipment

A swimming pool and a life vest for each athlete

Setup

Under the supervision of an adult who knows how to swim, athletes participate in the deep end of a swimming pool.

Execution

Athletes run in the deep end of the pool (refer to the tips on page 84 at the beginning of the chapter). Athletes should attempt to increase the total amount of time they can run without stopping by timing each attempt. Athletes make six attempts with a 60-second rest between each interval for the first session. Increase the number of intervals for each subsequent session. The degree of difficulty can eventually be increased by asking the athlete to run for a set continuous period of time (e.g., 10, 15, or 20 minutes) with the addition of faster paced intervals (e.g., 15, 30, 45, and 60 seconds) over the course of the total continuous run.

Ultimate Frisbee

Age Range

8 to 14

Purpose

To increase athletes' overall stamina

Benefits

Athletes build the stamina they need to execute skills effectively toward the end of competitions or when they become fatigued over the course of competition. The game consists of constant participant movement running forward and backward, quickly changing direction, and stopping and starting.

Equipment

A Frisbee, one vest per athlete (vests should be two different colors to distinguish teams)

Setup

The drill requires a playing field, either about 30 yards by 15 yards or about 70 yards by 40 yards, depending on the number of players.

Execution

The game can be played with either small (3 on 3) or larger groups (7 on 7). A 3-on-3 game should be played on a 30 × 15 yard field, and a 7-on-7 game should be played on a 70 × 40 yard field. The objective is to score by catching a Frisbee in a designated end zone, as in football. All athletes are involved and divided onto offense and defense teams; there are no designated positions. The Frisbee can move in any direction around the field, and play is continuous. Change of possession occurs when the Frisbee is thrown out of bounds, is dropped by the offense, is deflected by a defender to the ground, or after a score. When a change of possession occurs, the defense immediately goes on offense and begins play at the spot where the Frisbee was dropped, thrown out of bounds, or scored in the end zone. Players may take two steps after receiving the Frisbee and can transfer it only by throwing it to a teammate. Games can be any length, but we recommend two seven-minute halves. The objective is to keep everyone moving, so divide your group into an even number of teams and allow them all to play at the same time on different playing areas.

Sport-Specific Drill

DRILL 6.8
Baseball Stamina

Age Range

10 to 14

Purpose

To increase athletes' overall stamina

Benefits

Many youth baseball programs do not spend a lot of time on conditioning because of time constraints and the need to develop fundamentals. This drill focuses on both developing stamina and practicing basic baseball skills. The objective is to get all players moving—fielding balls on the ground and in the air, quickly moving the ball around, getting into position, collecting the ball before setting up and feeding to a teammate, and executing accurate long and short throws.

Equipment

A baseball glove for each player, a tennis ball, two baseball rebounders with 18-inch square targets (a tightly strung net with a target that allows balls to rebound back into the field of play), four cones or flat dots, chalk

Setup

In an area about 60 yards by 30 yards, place one baseball rebounder at each end of a field marked off with cones or flat dots. Mark off with chalk a line across the center of the field and two additional lines across the field 10 yards out from each rebounder and parallel to the center line. Also mark one line across each net's goal line across the width of the field (see diagram of field setup).

Execution

There are nine players per team who play the entire field of play, similar to soccer. The objective is to score by throwing a tennis ball directly into the rebounder, which serves as a goal. Bouncing the ball into the rebounder is not allowed. One point is awarded for hitting the goal; 3 points are awarded if the ball hits the goal's target.

When a team is on offense and has the ball in their offensive scoring zone (the area across the midfield point of the field where the opponent's goal is located between the midfield line and the line that crosses the field parallel to the goal line), the only way to pass the ball is by throwing a ground ball to a teammate. Once a player on offense receives the ball, he or she may take only four steps before passing to another teammate or throwing on goal. No player may position or make a play in the "dead zone" marked 10 yards out from each goal and across the entire field (see diagram). However, one offensive player is allowed to go behind the goal or goal line at a time in order to set up a play in their zone. Because this player must pass through the dead zone, he or she cannot stop or hesitate in his or her team's offensive zone; he or she must travel directly into the zone located behind the opponent's goal and remain there unless choosing to move back out into the offensive scoring zone (the area marked 10 yards out from the goal line out to midfield and 40 yards across the field). No other offensive player may move into the area behind their opponent's net until their teammate returns across the 10-yard line.

Offensive players may pass the ball by throwing to a teammate in the zone behind the goal or goal line; this is the only time a thrown pass in the air is allowed past midfield when a team is on offense. When play originates from inside the offensive side of the field, at least one ground ball pass must successfully be made before a throw on goal is allowed. The only exception is a pass coming from behind the net, which can be thrown in the air, caught, and thrown on goal.

Defenders attempt to intercept the balls on the ground or in the air by catching them and transitioning the play into their offensive end of the field by throwing to a teammate. Defenders are not allowed to play goalie. A marked-off 12-foot perimeter (use chalk or flat dots) around each goal designates the area that no defender may enter at any time. When a team intercepts a ball, they are allowed to throw the ball in the air out of their defensive zone. Remember that each player can take only four steps after receiving the ball before passing or throwing on goal.

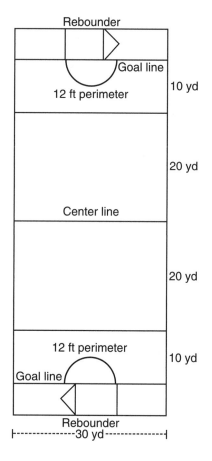

Change of possession occurs when the defense intercepts a pass, the ball travels out of bounds, or the offense scores. If there is a struggle for the ball between an offensive and defensive player, play is stopped, and the ball is awarded to the defense. Play resumes immediately after receiving possession of the ball at the spot where the last play ended. Games should last 14 minutes; teams switch sides at the 7-minute mark.

Football Stamina

Age Range

10 to 14

Purpose

To increase athletes' overall stamina

Benefits

Football practices are often difficult because of the amount of contact that takes place combined with the burden of wearing heavy equipment. Add heat and humidity, and many players are extremely fatigued by the end of a game. This drill works on conditioning for football and also focuses on performing skills when fatigued. The drill incorporates the passion kids have for video games while encouraging them to get outside and imitate the moves they witness on screen. Go to the Web site at www.nflstreetunplugged.com to find out where you can sign up to play in a national NFL Street Unplugged tour event.

Equipment

You'll need a football (intermediate size for 10- to 12-year-olds, regulation high school size for 13- and 14-year-olds), a stopwatch, and 12 cones. Optional equipment includes a Sony PSP video game player and EA Sport's NFL Street 3 video game.

Setup

In an area about 25 yards by 15 yards, use four cones to mark one end zone. Only one end zone is needed in this game. Use the remaining eight cones to mark each sideline, placing cones about 5 yards apart.

Execution

This game allows athletes to combine creative on-field play with NFL Street video game skills. Style points are awarded for skills such as one-handed receptions and behind-the-back catches.

Teams of three play with the objective of scoring or preventing as many trick plays as possible in the field of play or end zone. On-field scores are combined with on-site NFL Street video game scores to determine a winner.

There are three players per team; three play when on offense (quarterback and two wide receivers) and two play when on defense (two defensive backs). The third player sits out when his or her team is on defense and plays the video game on the portable handheld device.

Teams score points by either scoring touchdowns or by executing trick plays on the field. Players can choose from an array of tricks to earn points, and tricks are worth more points in the end zone than on the field. Style points can be combined on one play. For example, a diving catch in the end zone from a behind-the-back throw for a touchdown scores additional points. Style points are awarded based on the following scoring system:

	On field	In end zone
Between-the-legs reception *(a)*	30,000	50,000
Behind-the-back catch *(b)*	20,000	30,000
Between-the-legs throw with reception *(c)*	20,000	30,000
Behind-the-back throw with reception	10,000	20,000
One-handed reception *(d)*	10,000	20,000
Running figure-8s between legs	5,000	
Diving catch *(e)*	1,000	2,000
Successful tip to teammate	1,000	2,000
One-handed trap *(f)*	1,000	2,000
Touchdown	1,000	

Stamina and conditioning play a primary role in this game because each team plays five consecutive four-minute games of nonstop competition. Games consist of two consecutive minutes on offense, followed by two consecutive minutes on defense. The ball is never turned over to the defense during these two minutes. Touchdowns, interceptions, and fumbles are automatic dead balls, and play immediately begins again back at the 20-yard line.

Look for a complete explanation and video presentation of this game at www.nflstreetunplugged.com.

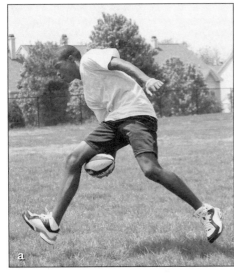

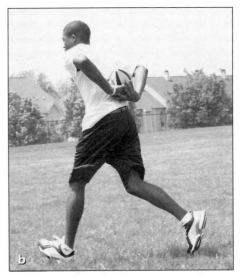

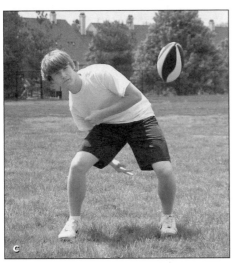

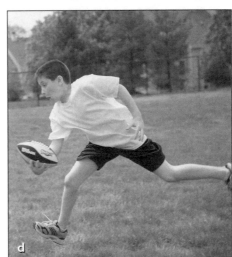

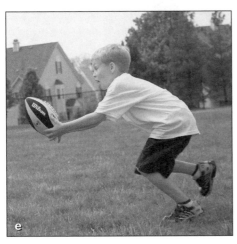

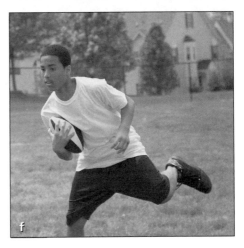

CHAPTER 7

Increase Strength

Athletes work on developing strength to improve their physical force or power. Strength is used in many different ways in different sports. A baseball player relies on strength for throwing with velocity and distance and to generate bat speed. Soccer players need strength when warding off an opponent as they fight for possession of a ball and to generate leg speed and power to kick with velocity and distance. Hockey players use their strength to knock their opponent off the puck, to skate with explosive power, to increase and maintain speed, and to shoot with maximum velocity.

As athletes mature into puberty, strength becomes a larger factor in some sports. For example, in baseball, when first developing hitting skills, bat speed plays a minor role compared to the importance of making contact with the ball. It's not until athletes begin to mature (around the ages of 12 to 14) and have experienced consistent improvement in making contact while batting that they should begin to focus on bat speed and power. In football, between the ages of 8 to 13 it's much more important to develop the fundamentals and techniques of blocking and tackling before shifting focus to developing the strength necessary to play at the upper levels.

Kids naturally build functional strength through their participation in activities and sports. Athletes between the ages of 8 and 12 will experience faster results and success with all other athletic elements discussed in this book than they will with strength. This is mainly because until puberty occurs, muscle strength develops at a much slower rate than after puberty. This doesn't imply that strength training should be ignored at early ages but that it should be done differently by age group.

Unfortunately, when many people think of strength training they automatically associate it with weight training. But because prepubescent kids make little to no progress in strength gains through weight training, there's no need to involve any type of weight equipment when working with the 8- to 12-year-old age groups—which should be fine with them because weight training is not a fun activity (at least not for most kids), and fun should be the key factor at this stage of development. Another reason to avoid weight training at young ages is that injury risk is much greater because of the undeveloped skeletal and muscular structures.

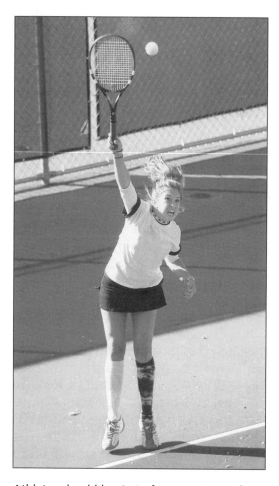

Athletes should begin to focus on strength and power once they have physically matured and are proficient in the fundamental techniques of their sport-specific skills.

For athletes from 8 to 12 years old, we'll focus primarily on continuing the development of natural strength through simple drills to support basic movement executions through proper technique. Most of this type of strength training occurs during play. Kids naturally develop strength through playing games and sports. When possible, mix fun strength-training competitions and drills into other forms of training and games (such as the strength obstacle course at the end of this chapter). Doing so deemphasizes the overall stress that strength training can place on a young body and allows for a more diverse training experience.

As children mature (12 years and older), their training will involve weight-training routines. After the age of 12, athletes should slowly accustom themselves to the use of free weights. But remember that weight training can be detrimental to athletes if they are not properly monitored and taught to lift properly. Be sure that athletes just beginning to weight train focus on proper lifting techniques and safety precautions before advancing to lifting significant weight. Strength training should support and enhance all of an athlete's movement training (agility, balance, coordination, flexibility, speed, and stamina); it should not be used primarily to build body mass and personal bests in bench pressing and squats. This can lead to a focus on how big or defined they can become rather than developing themselves as athletes and enhancing their sport skills. This training should also be supplemented with continually changing creative play options to refresh the training experience. Because weight training involves particular techniques that are vital to success, we recommend referring to *Weight Training Fundamentals* by David Sandler (Human Kinetics, 2003).

The following drills work separate muscle groups throughout the body with no focus placed on a particular body part or region. We believe that for this age group, this method best develops the strength of the child for multiple sports and athletic functions. Every drill and competition in this chapter plays an important role in preparing and strengthening the body to move with increased effectiveness and power.

DRILL 7.1
Forward and Backward Crawls

Age Range

8 to 14

Purpose

To improve strength in the arms, shoulders, legs, and core (abdominals, obliques, and lower back)

Benefits

Athletes experience a complete strength drill that develops the upper, lower, and core portions of the body that are vital for a majority of team sports, including baseball, basketball, football, hockey, and lacrosse.

Equipment

Four cones

Setup

Place two cones seven yards apart for one course; for a second course, place four cones in a diamond shape with five yards between each cone.

Execution

This drill is an expanded push-up type routine. Over four progressions the degree of difficulty increases and the age range narrows down to 11 to 14 years. Each progression involves both forward and backward crawls. In a forward crawl (a), athletes face the ground, placing both hands on the ground and using them to move their entire bodies forward. Athletes must also get up on their toes and drive their legs forward by alternating steps with the feet. Basically this is a forward walk with only hands and feet touching the ground.

In the backward crawl (b), each athlete places both hands on the ground, with the torso and head faceup and with the back facing the ground. Athletes must keep all body parts except for hands and feet elevated off the ground while moving backward. They move backward by alternating the movement of hands and feet in a backward direction.

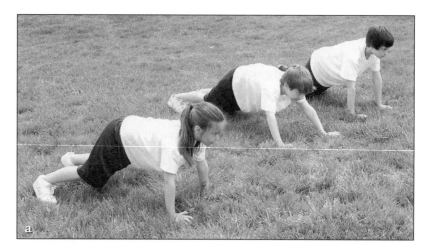

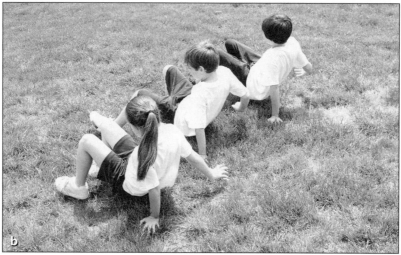

Progression 1

On a grass or turf field or court place two cones seven yards apart. Begin by starting athletes at one cone and asking them to execute a forward crawl to the next cone seven yards away. As athletes approach the cone, have them switch from a forward crawl to a backward crawl before fully making the turn around the cone. The athlete then returns to the starting cone seven yards away using a backward crawl.

Competition

Measure how long it takes for each athlete to crawl from one cone to the next and back.

Progression 2

Start athletes on the goal line of a football field and have them travel as far as they can in a forward crawl before falling to the ground.

Measure the distance covered by each athlete before he or she falls to the ground.

Progression 3

Place four cones five yards apart in a diamond shape on the ground (see diagram). Athletes begin by crawling forward from cone A to cone B (about five yards); they circle cone B with a 360-degree turn before switching to a backward crawl and moving to cone C; they circle cone C with a 360-degree turn before switching back to a forward crawl to cone D; they then circle and switch to a backward crawl and return to cone A.

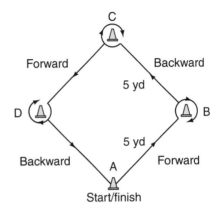

Competition

Record how many times athletes can travel around the course before falling to the ground. They receive 4 points for every successful lap before falling to the ground; they get 1 point for every cone reached in an unfinished lap.

Progression 4

For kids 11 to 12 years old, increase the level of difficulty by requiring each athlete to execute 10 push-ups after completing a 360-degree turn around each cone.

Competition

Record how many times athletes can travel around the course before falling to the ground. Athletes receive 4 points for every successful lap before falling to the ground; they get 1 point for every cone reached in an unfinished lap and half a point for every fully executed push-up.

DRILL 7.2
Fitness Tube

Age Range

8 to 14

Purpose

To improve total body strength

Benefits

This is a total body strength drill that develops the shoulders, arms, legs, and core.

Equipment

Exercise tubing (begin with light-resistance tubing for all ages and advance the 10- to 14-year-olds to medium resistance over time)

Setup

Perform this drill on a flat surface indoors or outdoors near a pole or tree.

Execution

This drill is composed of seven different exercises, each focusing on a separate body part. It's important that the athlete feel the muscle that's being worked on during the drill.

Shoulders

The athlete finds the middle of the tubing and places it on the ground with both feet standing on the midpoint. He or she holds each end of the tubing (through handles) with palms facing out at shoulder height and hands shoulder-width apart, knees slightly bent, and weight equally placed on both feet *(a)*. The back should be straight, and the head should be up looking straight ahead. The athlete performs the drill by pushing straight up into the air with both hands travel-ing directly over each shoulder at the same time until the elbows are nearly locked *(b)*. Athletes hold for one second, then slowly lower hands back to shoulder height and repeat 10 times. They should rest 90 seconds before beginning the next set of 10 repetitions. Have he or she complete three sets before moving to the next progression.

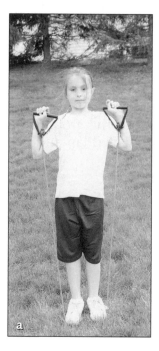
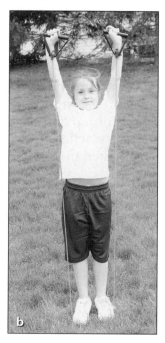

Triceps

Each athlete finds the middle of the tubing and places it on the ground with both feet standing on the midpoint. The athlete holds both hands together behind the neck and places the handles through the fingers of both hands. The tubing should run up the back of the athlete with the handles placed together 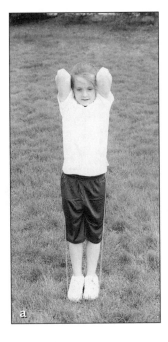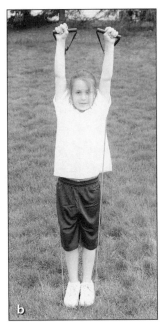 behind the head, elbows pointed forward and next to each ear, back straight, and head up looking straight ahead (a). Feet should be placed together with the knees slightly bent. The athlete performs the drill by pulling both hands straight up into the air directly over the head until the elbows lock (b), holding for one second, and then slowly returning the hands behind the head. Athletes should repeat 10 times, rest for 90 seconds, and then begin the next set of 10 repetitions. Have them complete three sets before moving to the next progression.

Biceps

Each athlete again finds the middle of the tubing and places it on the ground with both feet standing on the midpoint. The athlete holds each end of the tubing (through handles) with palms at hip level, hands shoulder-width apart, knees slightly bent, and weight equally placed on both feet (a). The back should be straight and head up looking straight ahead. The athlete performs the drill by pulling both handles at the same time until the hands reach shoulder height and are nearly touching each shoulder (b), holding for one second, and then slowly lowering the hands back to hip level. Athletes should repeat 10 times, rest 90 seconds, and then begin the next set of 10 repetitions. Have them complete three sets before moving to the next progression.

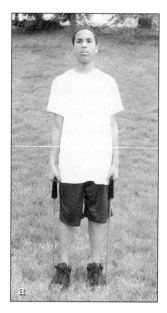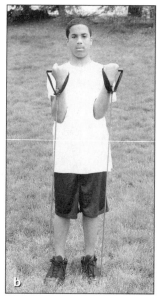

Forearms and Tops of Shoulders

Each athlete again finds the middle of the tubing and places it on the ground with both feet standing on the midpoint. The athlete holds each end of the tubing (through handles) with palms facing backward at hip level, hands shoulder-width apart, arms locked at the elbows, knees slightly bent, and weight equally placed on both feet *(a)*. The back should be straight and head should be up looking straight ahead. The athlete performs the drill by pulling both hands up at the same time with arms held straight out and elbows nearly locked until the

hands reach chest height *(b)*. After holding for one second, the athlete slowly lowers the hands back to hip level. Athletes should repeat 10 times, rest 90 seconds, and then begin the next set of 10 repetitions. Have them complete three sets before moving to the next progression.

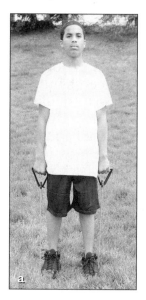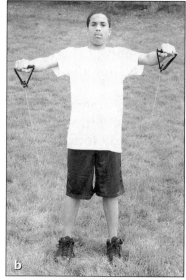

Chest

Each athlete loops the tubing around a pole or tree at chest height. The athlete holds each end of the tubing (through the handles) with palms facing out and forward. The back should be to the pole or tree. The athlete holds the tubing at chest level with arms extended out to each side and slightly bent at the elbows, knees slightly bent, and weight equally placed on both feet *(a)*. The back should be straight and head should be up looking straight ahead. The athlete performs the drill by pulling both hands together across the chest with arms straight out in front of the chest *(b)*. After holding for one second, the athlete slowly moves the hands back to each side of the chest. Athletes should repeat 10 times, rest 90 seconds, and then begin the next set of 10 repetitions. Have them complete three sets before moving to the next progression.

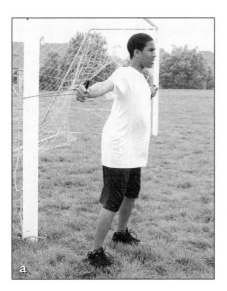 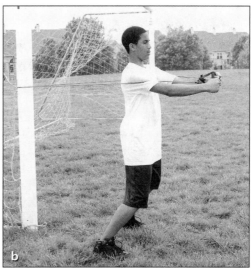

Arms and Shoulders

The athlete loops the middle of the tubing around a pole or tree at chest height with the back facing the tree or pole. He or she holds each end of the tubing (through the handles) with palms facing directly down, hands shoulder-width apart and placed on each side of the chest with elbows bent, knees slightly bent, and weight equally placed on both feet *(a)*. The back should be straight and head up looking straight ahead. The athlete performs the drill by punching each hand (one at a time) straight out *(b)* and back. Athletes should repeat 10 times, rest 90 seconds, and then begin the next set of 10 repetitions. Have them complete a total of three sets before moving to the next progression.

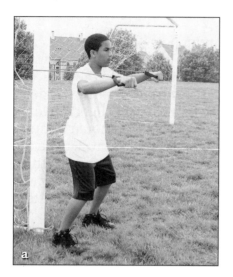 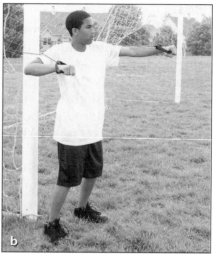

Thighs and Hip Flexors

Each athlete places the middle of the tubing around a pole or tree at ankle height with the back facing the tree or pole. The athlete places each foot through one end of the tubing (through the handles) with each foot facing straight ahead *(a)*. He or she places the feet shoulder-width apart and puts weight on the foot that's not pulling forward, keeping the back straight and head up. The athlete performs the drill by pulling the foot forward and away from the body, straight out and back, pulling until the knee is almost fully extended *(b)*. The athlete holds for one second and then slowly returns the foot to the starting position. Athletes should repeat 10 times before switching to the other foot. They should rest 90 seconds and then begin the next set of 10 repetitions. Have them complete three sets before moving to the next progression.

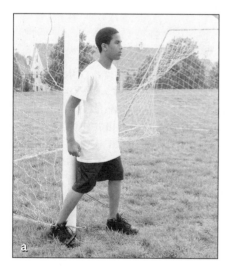 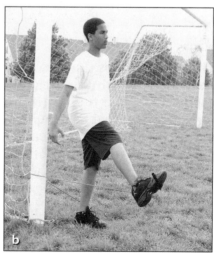

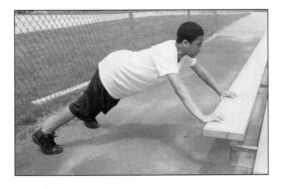

Competition

For all exercises, athletes can self-measure over the course of each session by recording the number of total reps per set (each additional rep earns 1 point) and the total number of additional sets (a minimum of 10 reps receives 10 points per additional set).

DRILL 7.3
Lateral Upper-Body Travel

Age Range

10 to 14

Purpose

To improve arm, shoulder, and core strength

Benefits

This drill improves strength throughout the upper body, which enhances power in baseball (throwing and batting), basketball (rebounding and warding off opponents), football (blocking, tackling, throwing, etc.), hockey (shooting, warding off opponents, checking, stick handling, etc.), lacrosse (shooting, passing, checking, warding off opponents), tennis (hitting, serving), and golf (swinging).

Equipment

A bench that's 8 to 12 feet long and 12 to 18 inches high

Setup

This drill can be done on a grass field or a basketball court.

Execution

These two progressions take the fully locked position of the elbows during the course of a push-up and challenge the athlete to move laterally in both directions across the length of an 8- to 12-foot bench.

Progression 1

Athletes place their hands on top of the bench about shoulder-width apart. They then walk their hands and feet laterally across the length of the bench, keeping their arms locked at the elbows, similar to the top of a fully extended push-up. Once they reach the

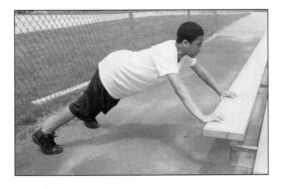

end of the bench, they return in the same way to the other end and continue back and forth until they can no longer support the weight of their bodies.

Competition

Measure how many times each athlete travels the full length of the bench without unlocking the elbows. They receive 1 point for the first pass from left to right and another for a pass right to left, 2 points for each second pass left to right and right to left, then 3 points for the third pass, and so on. Athletes can self-measure their progress by recording the total number of points they score in each session. (Note that athletes should do this drill no more than twice a week.)

Progression 2

Athletes place their hands on the ground shoulder-width apart and feet on the bench (also about shoulder-width apart). They then begin to walk their hands laterally across the ground while keeping both arms locked at the elbow, similar to the top of a fully extended push-up. They simultaneously move their feet laterally across the length of the bench. Once they reach the end of the bench, they return to the other side and repeat.

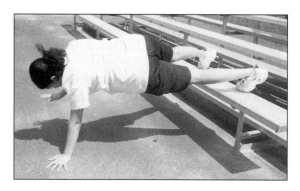

Competition

Measure how many times each athlete travels the full length of the bench without unlocking the elbows. They receive 1 point for the first pass from left to right and another for a pass right to left, 2 points for each second pass left to right and right to left, then 3 points for the third pass, and so on. Athletes can self-measure their progress by recording the total number of points they score in each session. (Note that athletes should do this drill no more than twice a week.)

DRILL 7.4
Diamond Push-Ups

Age Range

12 to 14 years

Purpose

To improve triceps, shoulder, and core strength

Benefits

This drill is both brief and extremely effective because of the intensity that is specifically focused on designated muscle groups.

Equipment

None

Setup

Conduct this drill on a grass field, tumbling mat, or carpet.

Execution

This drill is a variation of the traditional push-up that places more emphasis on the triceps, shoulders, abdomen, and backs of the legs. Each athlete begins by placing one hand on the ground and walking each hand out from the toes in front of the body until reaching five full hand lengths. The athlete then places the hands together with thumbs and pointer fingers touching, forming a diamond shape with the hands. The hips should form an upside-down V (a). The athlete attempts to touch the nose to the ground in the diamond space between both hands as many times as possible (b). This is a difficult drill and takes time to master and increase repetitions.

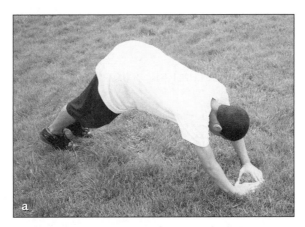

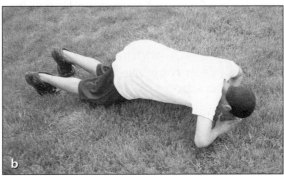

Competition

Measure the number of full repetitions (fully touching the ground with the nose), and ask each athlete to attempt to improve on that count over time.

DRILL 7.5

Lateral Bench Jumps

Age Range

8 to 14

Purpose

To improve arm, shoulder, hip flexor, and core strength

Benefits

This drill strengthens the shoulders while simultaneously developing power in the hip flexors (the muscles located on the upper outsides of the hips) through continuous explosive jumps and plyometric work, which is vital in improving speed.

Equipment

A bench that's 8 to 12 feet long and 12 to 18 inches high

Setup

Athletes perform this drill on a grass field, basketball court, track, or any flat stable surface. Several kids can do this drill at once at each end of the bench.

Execution

Each athlete begins by placing both feet on one side of the bench with each hand placed on each side of the bench; fingers should be grasping the outside edges of the bench. Athletes begin by leaping continuously from one side of the bench to the other for a count of 10 times. Arms are locked at the elbows and knees are slightly bent as they travel back and forth over the bench. They should land on the balls of the feet and immediately bounce off the ground and return to the other side of the bench. After 10 repetitions, athletes rest for one minute and then perform another set of 10 until they have done four to five total sets. Over time, athletes should build up to 20 reps per set.

Medicine Ball Throws

Age Range

8 to 14

Purpose

To improve strength in the arms, shoulders, legs, and core

Benefits

The use of a lightweight medicine ball is valuable in developing power and strength for all types of throwing, swinging, and rotating techniques. This is a total-body strength drill that develops the shoulders, arms, legs, and core.

Equipment

One medicine ball per athlete (1- to 2-pound ball for 8- to 11-year-olds; 4- to 6-pound ball for 12- to 14-year-olds)

Setup

Do this drill on a grass or turf football or soccer field.

Execution

Four progressions and three different throws are employed in this drill.

Progression 1

This progression builds strength in the upper back, chest, triceps, and forearms. The athlete begins by holding the ball against the chest with

elbows parallel to the ground and pointed straight out from each side of the body (a). Each hand is placed on the back side of the ball against the chest facing away from the body. The athlete executes the throw by stepping forward with one foot and pushing the ball out from the chest, keeping the back straight (b).

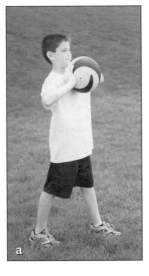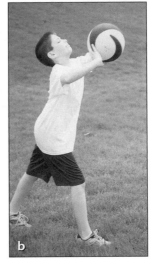

🏅 Competition

Measure the length of each throw along a straight line marked by a center line of chalk. Measure the distance from where the ball lands to the center line, and subtract that distance from the total distance of the throw. Athletes self-measure their progress over a period of time.

Progression 2

This progression involves a throw from each side of the body. This motion strengthens the baseball or tennis swing as well as the hip rotation for a golf swing. The athlete begins by grasping the ball with one hand on the top of the ball and one on the bottom *(a)*. The athlete's left side faces a designated point downfield (cone or chalk mark) for a right-side throw with the right hand on top and left hand placed on the bottom of the ball (reverse for the left side).

To execute the throw with the left shoulder facing a designated target downfield, the athlete extends both arms back about waist high, steps with the left foot laterally toward the downfield target, pivots with the back foot on the ball of the foot, rotates the hips (the right hip rotates until square with the designated target), and, with arms slightly bent and following, releases the ball as the arms catch up to the hips *(b)*. The throw continues with a complete follow-through that should finish with the left foot forward (with weight on the outside of the foot), the right foot completely turned toward the target (heel should lift and toes rotate toward target), and the hips square to the target.

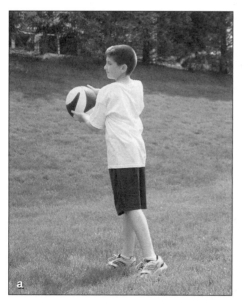
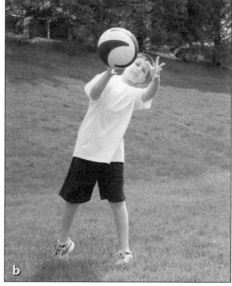

Competition

Measure the length of each throw along a straight line marked by a center line of chalk. Measure the distance from where the ball lands to the center line, and subtract that distance from the total distance of the throw. Athletes self-measure their progress over a period of time.

Progression 3

In this progression, the ball is thrown up and over the head to travel backward. The athlete squats with the ball placed between the legs and with hands grasping the ball on each side *(a)*. The athlete uses the legs to spring directly up off the ground, with the back straight and head looking forward, while simultaneously thrusting the arms up (slightly bent back) and releasing the ball just as the ball passes the forehead. The ball is thrown directly up and behind the athlete *(b)*. The object is to throw the ball backward as far as possible. Emphasize that athletes should be throwing for distance behind them and should not be throwing the ball directly up in the air. To avoid this, ask each athlete to step forward away from the throw immediately after releasing the ball.

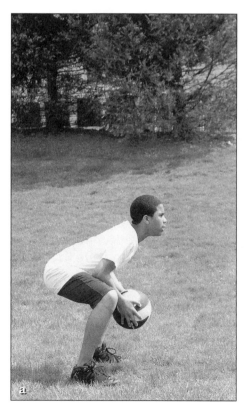 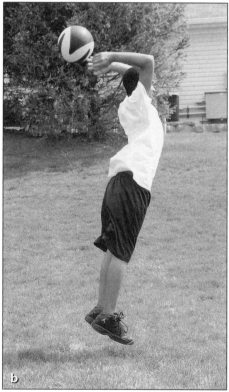

Measure the length of each throw along a straight line marked by a center line of chalk. Measure the distance from where the ball lands to the center line, and subtract that distance from the total distance of the throw. Athletes self-measure their progress over a period of time.

Progression 4

This relay race has been created for all three throwing techniques. Athletes begin by pairing off into groups of two. Each pair should have a one- or two-pound medicine ball per athlete. Athlete 1 throws the ball using the designated technique with athlete 2 standing next to him or her. Wherever the ball initially lands is the spot that athlete 2 must run to to make the next throw. After an athlete throws the ball, he or she immediately runs downfield as well to chase the next throw made by his or her partner. Each pair of athletes completes all three different throws as they travel up and down the field.

Sport-
Specific
Drill

DRILL 7.7
▰ Football Strength ▰

Age Range

12 to 14

Purpose

To improve overall power in the thighs, hips, and core

Benefits

This is a great drill to build strength while replicating football-specific situations, such as avoiding a tackle, blocking, and running with the ball through traffic.

Equipment

You'll need a football, six 6-inch hurdles, six 12-inch hurdles, one agility ladder, and an adjustable weighted vest. We recommend that athletes begin using a 5-pound vest or less before advancing to 10 pounds.

Setup

Run the drill on a flat surface indoors or outdoors. Arrange a course with a starting line and place six 6-inch hurdles five yards from the starting line in a row about two yards apart from each other. Place an agility ladder three yards to the left of the last 6-inch hurdle. Place six 12-inch hurdles to the left of the agility ladder about two yards apart in a row moving away from the starting line downfield (see diagram).

Execution

Each athlete runs with a football downfield five yards and over the six consecutive 6-inch hurdles before moving laterally through the agility ladder (the athlete faces downfield away from the starting line). The athlete then runs over the six consecutive 12-inch hurdles and on to the finish line marked five yards farther downfield. The athlete carries the ball the entire time.

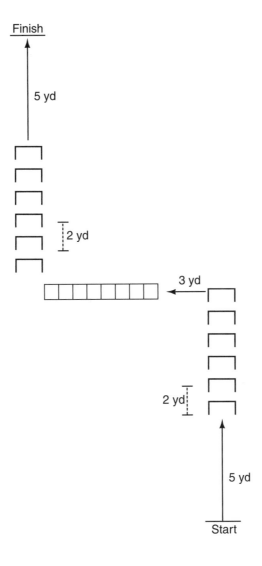

Basketball Strength

Age Range

10 to 14

Purpose

To improve overall strength and power for rebounding

Benefits

This drill builds strength and improves technique for rebounding in game situations.

Equipment

A two- to four-pound medicine ball

Setup

Run this drill on a basketball court or other comparable flat surface either indoors or outdoors. You'll need a solid wall that is at least 18 feet high adjacent to the court.

Execution

An athlete begins by having a partner throw a medicine ball against a wall at a height of at least 10 feet. The athlete catches the ball by keeping the arms fully extended over the head. The arms remain extended until they have possession for three seconds. The athlete then throws a chest pass as far as possible away from the wall.

Progression

Repeat the drill but require each athlete to keep the arms and ball fully extended for three seconds followed by an overhead pass as far as possible away from the wall.

CHAPTER 8

Maximize Speed

For our purposes, speed can be defined as the rate at which athletes move and also how quickly they react to a stimulus that causes a change in direction. Speed makes the difference in many athletic competitions. At any level of play of baseball, basketball, tennis, and many other sports, the team or individual that is faster has a sizeable advantage. Athletes use speed to get to their maximum rate of movement and then attempt to keep that pace as long as possible, or until a particular task is complete. We often witness the importance of speed as a midfielder chases a soccer ball downfield, a baseball player runs the bases, a basketball guard breaks for the basket, or a wide receiver sprints toward the end zone after a reception.

Each of these scenarios illustrates the importance of speed, but interestingly not one of them is executed or measured in the same way. The use of speed differs by sport and position within a sport. Different athletes might need to achieve maximum speed in shorter or longer distances or be able to hold that maximum speed for longer amounts of time. Some athletes might be starting from a stationary position and others from a moving position; they might have to react to different situations as quickly as possible. Rarely do you see athletes use speed in only one direction; more often it's paired with a rapid change in direction and incorporates agility (which we'll discuss in chapter 9). Clearly, it's important that we develop speed for numerous situations in sports.

Speed can also be measured in many ways. In this chapter we'll focus on two forms of speed: the speed of movement, or the time it takes to cover a specific distance, and the speed of reaction, or how quickly an athlete can respond to a specific stimuli, such as a sound, visual image, or touch. We'll first explain how to develop and increase a young athlete's overall running and reaction speed, and then we'll focus on how to apply speed of reaction to numerous athletic functions.

Nearly all athletes, naturally fast or not, can improve their speed, and this improvement almost always leads to improved all-around athletic performance. To improve a young athlete's speed, we must first teach the proper techniques involved in running. Proper running form and overall performance efficiency are essential for athletes to improve speed.

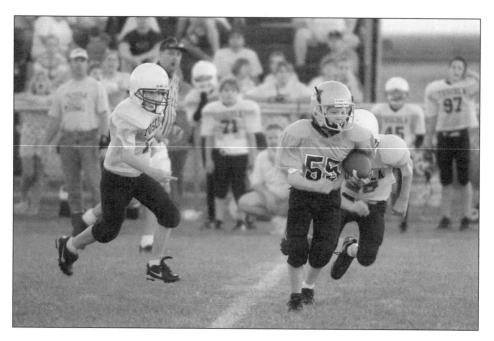

Speed allows athletes to outpace their opponents and to efficiently react to stimuli that require a quick change of direction.

If athletes learn to run properly, they'll have more energy and stamina throughout their sport performances.

One of the most overlooked elements in running is arm movement. Young athletes often run with their arms flailing in different directions. Watch a basketball or soccer game and you'll witness young players running with arms moving across their bodies, elbows pointing to each side. Rather than relaxed cupped hands, you might see something like a full windmill, arms rotating like airplane propellers. But who can blame kids for running this way when they've never been shown the proper way to run?

It's never too early or too late to learn to run properly. Once they're taught proper running technique, athletes begin to experience faster overall times and increased stamina as a result of reduced energy waste. Nearly any athlete can benefit from form running and correcting slight flaws they can't detect themselves. The form-running drills in this chapter guide athletes through a series of exercises that focus on one body part at a time. The idea is to develop memory in each muscle or muscle group before combining the parts. Also included in the chapter are several individual competitions to allow athletes to self-measure overall progress.

Many other drills in this book can be used to increase running speed. Some of these can be found in the agility, strength, and stamina chapters. For example, the 30-Yard Athletic Slalom drill in chapter 9 (agility) prepares athletes for a range of athletic movements that must be made while running or skating in a variety of competitions. Remember that many of these athletic components are interrelated; you can't develop one element, such as speed, without affecting others, such as agility, flexibility, stamina, and strength.

Along with learning to run forward properly, it's also important for athletes to know how to backpedal, or run backward, efficiently. During many types of athletic competition athletes must backpedal, and the speed at which they can do so might be the difference between a victory and a loss. As with form running, it's important to practice the proper techniques of running backward. In this case, the best way to communicate proper technique is for athletes to observe it, either through an active demonstration or by watching a video, which you can find on www.youthevolutionsports.com. Unlike form running, athletes don't stand erect when running backward. If they did, they would likely lose their balance and fall. Proper posture for backpedaling is with the waist slightly bent and shoulders positioned over the knees. The head should be looking forward.

Also important when athletes are backpedaling is how well they can react and transition to execute a movement in another direction. Athletes will often transition from a backpedal to a full forward run to pursue an opponent or the ball. For example, when a soccer defender is backpedaling as a ball-handler approaches, he or she must first determine and react to the ball-handler's first move to get by him or her by turning the hips in the correct direction and quickly transitioning into a position to run and stay with the opponent or take back possession of the ball. Similar situations arise for lacrosse defenders or for defensive backs in football. The transition from backpedaling to running is crucial because of the importance of not losing a step on your opponent or the possibility of regaining possession of the ball. Thus, the initial pivot and move are vital and should be practiced. This is a great example of how speed and agility skills combine in order to fully execute the most effective movements in an athletic competition. (For more details on backpedaling techniques and transitions, please visit www.youthevolutionsports.com.) This type of movement execution is common to most sports. Though every sport differs in its techniques for backpedaling and transitioning situations, drill 8.2 in this chapter introduce basic movements that build a foundation for becoming more accustomed to the movement. Proper form should always be used no matter the athletic situation to eliminate all wasted movement and maximize traveling from point A to point B as quickly as possible.

Competition involves frequent stops and starts, changes of direction, and maneuvering around defenders as quickly as possible. The speed of an athlete is often interrupted by an intentional knockdown or an unintentional fall. They must recover immediately by getting back up and proceeding with the play. Young athletes are often asked to perform these moves in competition without the advantage of practicing and preparing the body's muscle memory to take over when the time comes to actually execute. Athletes should practice movement changes to prepare themselves for competition. The drills and competitions in this chapter provide a great base to begin developing overall running and reactive speed. Many additional drills and competitions are available and will be continually updated on www.youthevolutionsports.com.

DRILL 8.1
Form Running

Age Range

8 to 14

Purpose

To improve an athlete's speed potential by correcting flaws in running form

Benefits

Without proper running form, athletes will never reach their optimal speed potential. Proper running form allows athletes to eliminate wasted movement, become more efficient, and travel faster in any direction. Athletes in any sport that requires running should work on proper running form. Six elements make up an athlete's running form, including arm movement, high knees, butt kicks, straight legs, bounding, and rapid leg turnover. This drill progressively works on each of these elements.

Equipment

Four cones, 10 12-inch hurdles

Setup

In an open space, form a 30-yard by 30-yard square with cones.

Execution

Athletes line up in a straight line between a pair of cones placed 30 yards apart. They perform each progression simultaneously by traveling in a straight line until they reach the next set of cones 30 yards downfield. As they reach the second set of cones, athletes stop and wait until everyone is once again ready to return to the original set of cones. Emphasize moving in a straight line and not straying into other athletes' invisible lanes.

Progression 1: Arm Movement

Athletes walk in a straight line for 30 yards, focusing on marching with arms bent 45 degrees at the elbows. The shoulder, not the elbow, should initiate the arm swing. Arms swing with elbows positioned

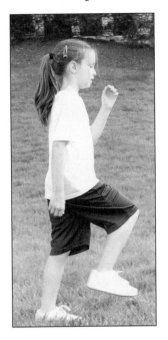

as close to the body as possible, moving in a straight line forward and back. To emphasize proper movement, ask athletes to imagine and feel their elbows shooting straight back as if at a target directly behind them. Arms should also move straight forward, with hands finishing the forward swing no higher than the nose. Arms should never cross in front of the body. Tell your athletes that they should see their hands only from the outside corners of their eyes, never directly in front of them. Hands should be gently cupped and relaxed, not clenched or flat with fingers straight. This prevents arms from tightening and losing their full range of motion during the arm swing. As athletes march forward, their heads and upper torsos should remain as still as possible with shoulders back, not hunched forward. Repeat four times.

Progression 2: High Knees

After they master proper arm movement, athletes perform four 30-yard marches incorporating high knees. This drill exaggerates lifting the knees in comparison to a normal running stride to train athletes to drive their bodies forward. Without generating power in the hip flexors (the upper and outer muscles of the hips), athletes can't move at optimal speed. The knee-lift is basically a focal point that we ask each athlete to execute in order to train and build the overall forward running stride. Ask athletes to try to get their knees as high as their chests; this helps make the point that knees must drive straight up. The calf muscle is folded against the hamstrings, and the thigh is parallel to the ground. As each foot hits the ground, toes should point up, which allows the legs to explode into the next stride. Each stride length should be

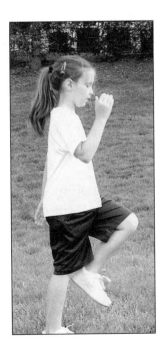

short and conducted slowly. The faster the arms move, the faster the legs will move. It's important that athletes perform this drill slowly with many repetitions of rapid knee-lifts. After they complete four 30-yard walks, have them do four 30-yard jogs with high knees. Remind them that this drill is a jog and should be done slowly. Emphasize that this is not a race but rather an opportunity to focus on how high they can lift their knees.

Progression 3: Butt Kicks

This is another exaggerated movement that trains the legs to complete the full range of motion during the running stride. To get a full rotation of each leg around as quickly as possible, athletes cannot forget the backside of the leg's rotation. They can't run fast without getting their back heels as high as possible. This progression isolates, replicates, and exaggerates that movement in order to create muscle memory when all the pieces of the running form are put together. Don't be concerned if athletes can't touch their butts with their heels during this drill. The primary goal is to get the heel as high as possible to create full range of motion.

Athletes complete four 30-yard jogs with an emphasis on kicking their heels back to their butts. To get the knee up and driving forward, the thigh remains parallel to the ground, with the heel nearly touching the butt. (This might seem to contradict previous instruction to get the knees as high as possible, but remember that each drill emphasizes one particular aspect of the running stride. The knee-lift was not the actual stride used during a run.)

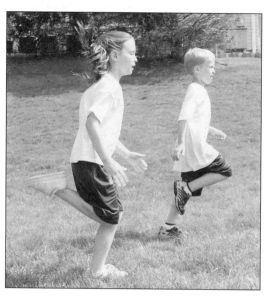

Athletes should drive each leg back to the ground rapidly after touching their butts, causing the feet to pull the ground backward as the body explodes forward. Ask them to feel their toes pulling toward their shins each time their feet contact the ground; this activates the calf muscle and helps the body propel forward by pushing against the ground. The positioning of the toes toward the shin on each stride pulls each foot through faster, thereby increasing running speed.

Progression 4: Straight Legs

This progression develops the feel for pulling back against the running surface, which is essential in propelling the body forward. Athletes begin by walking in a straight line, keeping legs straight with no knee bend. They swing each leg forward *from the hip* and quickly back to the ground. Remind them to keep their toes up to get their feet off the ground faster; keeping toes up is how they produce the counterforce that propels them forward. They should begin by executing two 30-yard walks. When they feel comfortable and can execute the drill properly, progress them to four 30-yard jogs using the same technique. By moving from a walk to a jog, they begin to feel the greater backward pulling force of each foot.

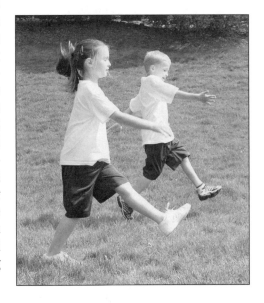

Progression 5: Bounding

This progression emphasizes and strengthens the body's ability to explode forward. It incorporates all the components of form running while strengthening the athlete. The best way to explain this drill, and the most successful way we've found to teach it, is to ask athletes to visualize jumping over successive puddles without stopping. The athlete should drive forward with the right knee, using the left leg to thrust off the ground (toes up) for distance. He or she lands on the right foot and immediately thrusts off the ground with the same foot (toes up), this time driving the left knee forward. This continues throughout the drill.

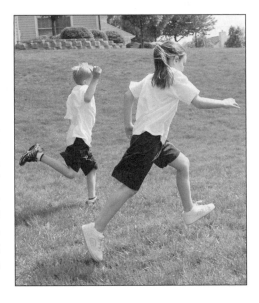

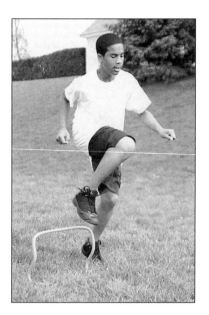

Progression 6: Rapid Leg Turnover

Set up 6 to 10 12-inch hurdles about 10 feet apart. Start the drill by asking each athlete to jog forward and step over each hurdle with the right foot while thrusting the left leg rapidly over each hurdle, using the same butt-kick action used in an earlier progression. Then repeat with the right leg. Progress athletes by moving hurdles closer together for quicker execution. Repeat five to eight times.

DRILL 8.2
Backward Speed

Age Range

8 to 14

Purpose

To improve backpedaling speed by correcting flaws in running form

Benefits

Proper running form allows athletes to eliminate all wasted movements so that they become more efficient and can travel faster in any direction. Backpedaling is an essential skill used in most sports, but each sport incorporates different techniques in order to execute the skill properly. This drill emphasizes a general approach, or a foundation to backpedaling. Individual sport applications can be found at www.youthevolutionsports.com.

Equipment

Four cones

Setup

Form a 30-yard by 30-yard square with cones.

Execution

Athletes line up in a straight line between a pair of cones placed 30 yards apart. They backpedal for four sets of 30 yards, taking short quick steps while keeping a fast tempo with the arms. The arm-swing technique should be identical to running forward but is now moving in the opposite direction. Each athlete's head should be up, looking straight ahead (many athletes tend to look down at their feet). The body should have a slight bend at the waist, keeping the feet close together and underneath the athlete's body (to remain stable and prevent the athlete from falling); otherwise, a long stride will slow the athlete by creating an unstable position. Emphasize moving in a straight line and not straying into other athletes' invisible lanes.

DRILL 8.3
Change of Direction

Age Range

8 to 14

Purpose

To improve on how quickly athletes can change direction during competition

Benefits

Much of the time playing a sport is spent changing direction. This drill works on changing direction from a straight-on run to taking angles to a spot on a field or court. Athletes will experience this type of change of direction in basketball, football, lacrosse, soccer, and tennis.

Equipment

Six cones, a stopwatch

Setup

Set up one cone as a starting line, and place cone A 10 yards downfield from the starting cone. Place cone B 10 yards directly to the right of cone A, and place cone C 10 yards to the left of cone A. Place two additional cones at 45-degree angles downfield from cone A, one to the right and one to the left.

Execution

There are two progressions. The first emphasizes the proper technique used to change direction as quickly as possible. The second focuses on reaction, which is the primary reason athletes change direction during competition.

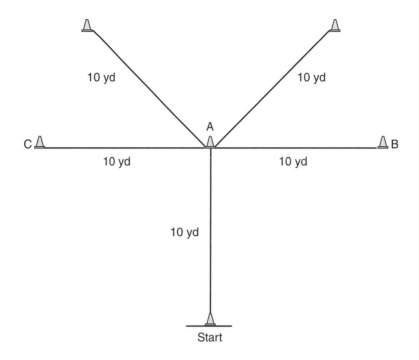

10 yd   10 yd

C   A   B
    10 yd   10 yd

10 yd

Start

Progression 1

An athlete runs at half-speed from the starting line to cone A, plants the left foot, and runs at half-speed directly to cone B. Athletes should plant their left feet for all runs to their right; they plant their right feet for all runs to their left. They repeat half-speed repetitions to all four cones until they can consistently cut with the correct foot and feel comfortable executing the drill. To keep from losing speed when changing direction, it is important to point out that the leg that cuts should not dip at the hip; it should extend and cut.

Competition

Measure the competition by timing athletes' full-speed runs from the starting line to cone A and then immediately to another cone. Time each run to each designated cone, and establish a personal-best time to each cone over the course of three attempts. After athletes' personal bests are established for each cone, award them 1 point for each quarter-second they can run under their personal-best time for each cone.

Progression 2

Progress the drill by adding the element of reaction speed. An athlete's change in direction is often caused by reacting as quickly as possible to a defender, the ball, or a teammate. This progression works on both speed of movement and speed of reaction. Start by having a partner stand five yards downfield from cone A with the responsibility of pointing to a particular cone as soon as the athlete reaches cone A. The athlete begins at the starting line and runs full speed to cone A. Just as he or she approaches cone A, the partner points to one of the other four cones; the athlete then responds by running to the cone the partner points to.

Competition

Measure the competition by timing the athlete's full-speed run from the starting line to cone A and then to the other cone. Time each run to each designated cone, and establish a personal-best time over the course of three attempts. After athletes' personal bests are established, award them 2 points for each quarter-second they can run under their personal-best time from cone to cone.

DRILL 8.4
Multiple Speed Moves

Age Range

8 to 14

Purpose

To increase speed when changing direction from a lateral to a forward movement

Benefits

Many kids never get the opportunity to experience or work on moving laterally then exploding into a forward sprint in pursuit of an opponent, ball, or puck. This type of movement is executed very often during athletic competitions, yet it is rarely focused on in training. The more effectively an athlete can move laterally and transition into an explosive forward movement, the better prepared and effective he or she will be in competition.

Equipment

Nine cones

Setup

Place eight cones in a circle with a ninth cone in the center of the circle (cone A). The eight cones are placed five yards from cone A, with two placed at 180 degrees (B and F) to cone A, one cone (C) placed at 45 degrees, one cone (D) placed at 90 degrees, one cone (E) at 135 degrees, another cone (G) at 225 degrees, one cone (H) at 270 degrees, and the final cone (I) at 315 degrees.

Execution

Athletes execute three progressions that incorporate forward, lateral, and backpedaling movements.

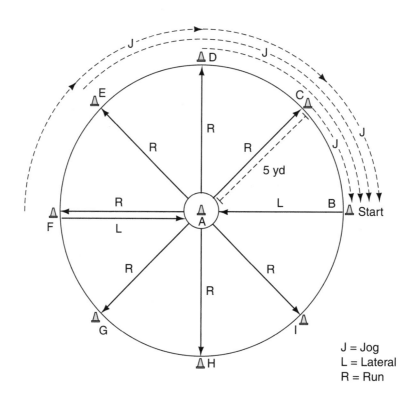

J = Jog
L = Lateral
R = Run

Progression 1

This first progression emphasizes transitioning from a lateral run to a full sprint in different directions. Athletes begin by facing in the direction of the top half of the circle, facing cones C, D, and E. The drill begins with a three-cone sequence: The athlete starts at cone B, moves laterally to touch cone A, and then immediately sprints at 45 degrees to touch cone C. The athlete then jogs clockwise from cone C back to touch cone B to begin the next three-cone sequence, moving laterally to touch cone A and then sprinting at 90 degrees to touch cone D. This drill continues counterclockwise around the circle with lateral and forward sprints to touch each of the remaining cones followed by a clockwise jog around to begin each new three-cone sequence back at cone B.

After completing lateral-to-forward sprints to every cone around the circle, the drill continues with three-cone sequences starting from cone F. The athlete moves laterally left to right from cone F to cone A and then sprints to touch cone C. This is followed by a jog counterclockwise back to touch cone F. This continues until every cone has been touched on the perimeter, completing the entire circle.

Competition

This self-measuring competition can be conducted by clocking the time it takes athletes to execute each sequence (e.g., the lateral move from cone B to touch cone A followed by sprinting to cone C). A total of eight timed sequences are recorded counterclockwise and another eight in a clockwise direction. Add all three-cone-sequence times together to establish a personal best. To measure progress, an athlete is then assigned one point for every quarter of a second recorded under the athlete's personal best. A new personal best is posted every time an improved time is recorded.

Progression 2

An athlete starts with his or her back to the course at cone H. The athlete completes each sequence by backpedaling five yards, touching cone A, and then immediately sprinting and touching a cone five yards away in any of the multiple directions (45, 90, 135, 180 degrees, etc.) around the perimeter of the circle. The athlete repeats the sequence until every cone has been touched, always jogging clockwise back to cone H after each sequence.

Competition

Like the last one, this is a self-measuring competition that clocks each sequence and allows for only the correct execution of backpedaling and turning to sprint through to touch the designated cone. Record a total of eight timed sequences; add all three-cone-sequence times together to establish a personal best. An athlete is then assigned one point for every quarter of a second recorded under the athlete's personal best. A new personal best is posted every time an improved time is recorded.

Progression 3

This progression combines the multiple movements of lateral running, backpedaling, and forward running as a means to test overall agility. This progression involves a new setup with two agility ladders and five cones (see diagram on next page). An athlete starts at cone A and laterally runs left to right through two agility ladders, placing only one foot in each square and keeping hips and shoulders square until reaching cone B. Between agility ladders, the athlete must keep running laterally. The athlete then continues back from cone B laterally right to left through one ladder to cone C. The athlete then immediately backpedals from cone C to cone D, runs from cone D to cone C, turns and backpedals from cone C to cone E, and then finishes by running from cone E to cone C.

Competition

Time how long it takes athletes to execute the course. Each athlete must take only one lateral step per agility ladder square. They must also touch each cone before executing the next move. After a series of four timed runs, take the best time and assign that as the athlete's personal best. All runs thereafter are assigned one point for every quarter of a second recorded under the athlete's personal best. A new personal best is posted every time an improved time is recorded.

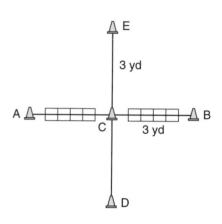

Slalom Dash

Age Range

8 to 14

Purpose

To improve on how quickly athletes can change direction during competition

Benefits

Downfield speed in its purest form is rarely a factor in most sports. Much more often athletes are faced with situations in which they must adjust while attempting to get from point A to point B as quickly as possible. This slalom dash course simulates movements an athlete uses when pursuing an elusive opponent or when trying to beat an opponent to a particular spot on the field.

Equipment

Five cones, a stopwatch

Setup

Set up cone A as a starting line and cone B 10 yards upfield from cone A. Place cone C 5 yards downfield from cone B (back toward the direction of cone A) and 5 yards to the left of cone B. Place cone D 5 yards back upfield and 5 yards to the left of cone C. Place the final cone (E) 10 yards downfield from cone D.

Execution

An athlete begins by running full speed from cone A to cone B, where he or she plants the right foot and dips the left shoulder around the right side of the cone before sprinting back downfield to cone C, where the athlete plants the left foot and dips the right shoulder around the left side of the cone, and then sprints upfield to cone D. At cone D, he or she plants the right foot and dips the left shoulder around the right side of the cone and sprints to the finish at cone E. After completing the course, athletes restart, this time running the drill in the opposite direction. There is no direct penalty for planting or dipping with the wrong foot or shoulder, but point out that proper execution of the drill will reduce their overall time.

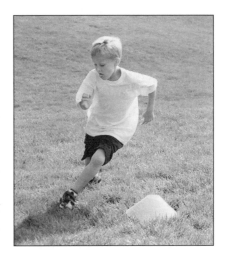

🏅 Competition

Measure the competition by timing athletes as they complete the course. After they have recorded times for five executions, take the fastest time and use it as the base. Award 1 point for every second recorded under the athlete's base time each time he or she runs the course.

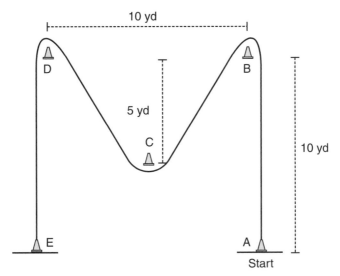

Competitive Speed

Age Range

8 to 14

Purpose

To improve an athlete's speed when faced with obstacles and competitive situations

Benefits

This drill helps athletes accustom themselves to perfect stops and starts, changes of direction, falls and recoveries, and maneuvers around defenders, all done as quickly as possible. The drill applies to movements in many sports, including baseball, basketball, hockey, lacrosse, soccer, and tennis.

Equipment

Nine cones, a stopwatch

Setup

Set up cone A as a starting line and place cone B 10 yards in front of cone A. Cone B becomes the center of a circle. Place the remaining cones in a circle as shown in the diagram.

Execution

There are two progressions. The first emphasizes proper technique for changing direction as quickly as possible. The second focuses on reaction, which is the primary reason athletes change direction during competition.

Progression 1

Each athlete begins at cone A and runs the complete course to each cone (A to B to C, A to B to D, and so on), planting with the correct foot and sprinting to the next designated cone. Athletes stop after each three-cone execution and start again at cone A for the next set of three cones.

Competition

Measure the competition by timing athletes as they run full speed from cone A to cone B and then on to another specific cone. Time each run from cone A to cone B to each perimeter cone and establish a personal-best time to each perimeter cone over the course of three attempts. After an athlete's personal best is established for each perimeter cone, award the athlete 1 point for each quarter-second under his or her personal-best time to each cone.

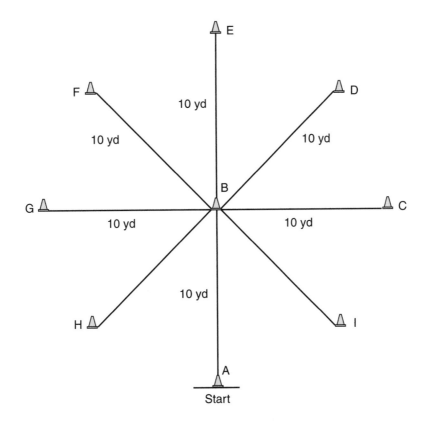

Progression 2

In this progression, athletes practice speed of movement and reaction. Repeat the first progression, but add someone standing at cone B pointing out which cone to run to just as the athlete arrives at cone B and plants to move to the next cone.

Competition

Establish a personal-best time in the same way as in the previous competition. After an athlete's personal best is established for each cone, award him or her 4 points for each quarter-second under his or her personal-best time to each cone.

DRILL 8.7
Speed From the Ground Up

Age Range

8 to 14

Purpose

To improve an athlete's speed when faced with numerous competitive situations

Benefits

This drill simulates reacting to different situations while on the ground and then transitioning that reaction into the maximum amount of speed to finish a play.

Equipment

Two cones, a stopwatch

Setup

Set up cone A as a starting line and cone B as a finish line 20 yards away.

Execution

Athletes start at cone A. Each athlete assumes a different starting position each time, including sitting facing the finish line or with his or her back to the finish line, lying down on the belly or back, and sitting cross-legged. On a signal, athletes launch into a full sprint to the finish line. Vary the signal each time, using sound (whistle, voice, hand clap), sight (hand signal), and touch (tap on the shoulder).

🏅 Competition

Each time the competition is conducted, athletes measure their progress and attempt to improve on each of their recorded times. Award 1 point to athletes for every quarter-second they shave off their personal-best time for each start position. This allows all athletes to self-measure their progress without comparing themselves to others.

Sport-
Specific
Drill

DRILL 8.8
Basketball Speed

Age Range

8 to 14

Purpose

To improve an athlete's basketball speed in different situations with a basketball

Benefits

This drill simulates gamelike situations in which speed is essential.

Equipment

Seven cones, a basketball, a basketball backboard, a stopwatch

Setup

Place cone A on a basketball court 60 feet from the backboard. Place two more cones (B and C) 10 feet apart from each other and 15 feet from cone A. Place two more cones (D and E) 10 feet apart from each other and 15 feet downcourt from cones B and C. Place the third and last set of cones (F and G) 10 feet apart from each other and 15 feet downcourt of cones D and E. This last pair of cones is 15 feet from the backboard.

Execution

An athlete sprints from cone A to cones B and C. When passing cones B and C, someone stationed at cones D and E drops a basketball from shoulder height onto the court. The athlete sprints to the ball, controls it, and dribbles around cones F and G left to right. This is followed immediately by dribbling toward the backboard, throwing the ball against the backboard, retrieving the ball, and dribbling around cones G and F left to right and then past cones E and D, which serve as the finish line.

🏅 Competition

Record how long it takes to finish the course. If cones F and G are missed, a penalty of three seconds per cone is added to the final time. Athletes measure their progress and attempt to beat their best time.

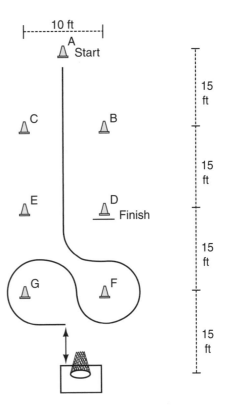

Soccer Speed

Age Range

8 to 14

Purpose

To improve an athlete's soccer speed with and without a soccer ball

Benefits

This drill simulates gamelike situations in soccer in which speed is essential.

Equipment

Eight cones, one soccer ball, two benches, six 12-inch minihurdles, a stopwatch

Setup

On a soccer field, place two cones about 10 feet apart at the midfield sideline (point A). Place two more cones 10 feet apart 20 yards downfield on the same sideline (point B). Place two benches on the ground with the ends of the seats facing the athlete as he or she runs down the field, one placed 10 yards off the sideline (point C) about 20 yards downfield from point B, and the second placed on the sideline another 5 yards downfield (point D). Place two cones 10 feet apart 50 yards from the starting area (point E). Set up six 12-inch minihurdles in a row in the opposite direction of the course about 3 yards apart (between points F and G). Place two cones at point H to designate the finish line of the course. One soccer ball is placed on the field at point B (see diagram).

Execution

An athlete sprints from point A to a soccer ball placed at point B. The athlete then dribbles the ball to point C, where he or she passes the ball against the bench, retrieves the ball (simulating a give-and-go), and dribbles toward point D, where once again the ball is passed against a bench, simulating another give-and-go. The athlete then continues to dribble downfield 5 yards to point E. This is followed by dribbling the ball to the next station on the same end line (point F) and then dribbling back in the opposite direction back upfield, jumping over six consecutive hurdles placed 3 yards apart and dribbling the ball under each hurdle. After clearing the sixth hurdle and successfully dribbling the ball straight through all hurdles, the athlete continues dribbling 10 yards to the finish at point H.

Competition

Record how long it takes each athlete to finish the 80-yard course. If a pass misses a bench, or the ball doesn't travel through all hurdles, apply a three-second penalty that is added to the athlete's time. Athletes measure their progress and attempt to beat their best time.

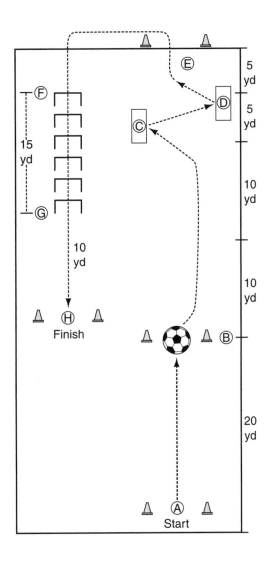

CHAPTER 9

Enhance Agility

Athletes with agility tend to be speedy and flexible and possess a combination of mental quickness, alertness, and intelligence. Agility is the core element that shapes all athletes. A basketball player relies on agility to move quickly and efficiently on the court. A football player uses agility in the basic movements of tackling and blocking. Agility is also important in the execution of highly skilled moves such as a wide receiver running a passing route, a quarterback dropping back to pass, or a defensive back covering a wide receiver, to name just a few. The game of soccer also requires a great deal of agility. In fact, agility plays a role in just about every interactive movement an athlete makes on a soccer field, whether with the ball, a teammate, an opponent, or all three at once.

To succeed in any sport, athletes must develop the most effective and efficient ways to move. Agility training is primarily about body awareness and establishing rhythm in an athlete's movements. The more aware athletes are of how their bodies feel when executing different movements at different speeds, the more success they'll experience in competition. This *feel*, also called muscle memory or muscle knowledge, is an actual rhythm the body creates to remember and react under different circumstances. (This concept was also explored in chapter 4.) Think of a young athlete playing in a soccer game. There are so many combinations of body movements that occur during the course of a game, from stop-and-go running, to cutting with one foot in one direction and immediately cutting back with the other foot, to running with the ball or passing to receive the ball, all while moving at various speeds in one smooth transition. Agility and coordination are closely connected, and agility training is an important precursor to developing coordination. Imagine sport-specific coordination skills such as a quarterback throwing on the run, a soccer player jumping and heading a soccer ball, or a hockey player skating full speed without missing a stride to take a shot on goal—none of these would be possible if athletes had not developed their agility.

As athletes develop their agility skills, they are also increasing their body awareness. Athletes with good agility don't have to think about what they're doing; instead, they instinctually execute with the body and mind. An agile running back in football avoids potential tacklers

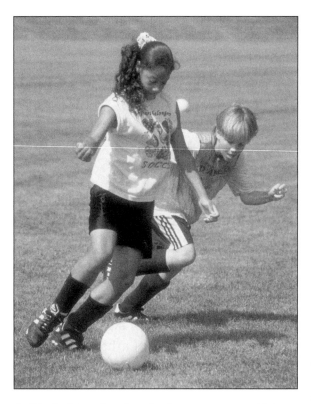

Agility training develops body awareness, which allows an athlete to perform sport-specific skills such as handling a soccer ball while simultaneously maneuvering around an opponent.

without thinking about those moves, yet he is subconsciously aware of what his body must do in order to react and execute those particular moves. A basketball player doesn't consciously make decisions to cut with the left foot to immediately move to the right around a defender. Agility training prepares the body to react and become comfortable moving in the most effective and efficient ways possible in order to make crucial plays and improve overall performance. All types of upper- and lower-body movements, either separate or synchronized, become second nature with agility training. The most complete and successful athlete cannot advance without continuing to develop this most vital physical element. Agility training develops athletes' creative abilities, allowing them to customize their athletic movements and develop their own style.

Some coaches combine agility training with overall conditioning, but this is not recommended. Agility skills are very important and deserve a singular focus. It's essential to allow the body to become familiar with specific body movements. After body movements have been adequately established under controlled circumstances, athletes may begin varying situations and increasing the complexity of movements under different conditions. For example, they might add endurance or the coordination of additional tasks, such as passing a football on the run or bulleting a throw to first base while sliding on the ground.

The earlier young athletes are exposed to agility training, the faster they'll experience improved overall performance. Of all the athletic elements, agility should be the most enjoyable for kids to learn because agility allows for creativity. No one athlete moves exactly the same as another, so every athlete must find his or her own most effective way to move. This is where athletes can develop their own styles. Top athletes such as Reggie Bush of the New Orleans Saints, Dwyane Wade of the Miami Heat, or Daisuke Matsuzaka of the Boston Red Sox all move in their own individual and creative ways. Agility training allows a young athlete to develop his or her own style in relation to body build and developing abilities. The drills in this chapter are fun yet challenging—to the point that kids want to continuously execute and perfect them.

DRILL 9.1
Body Awareness and Control

Age Range

8 to 14

Purpose

To improve body awareness and learn to control the body while moving

Benefits

Because of the nature of sport, most athletes are placed in situations during the free flow of competition in which they are turned around, twisted, or spun; they then must quickly orient themselves and react to the action around them. This drill trains the mind and body to work together to become quickly aware and to react.

Equipment

A chair or bench that stands at least 18 inches off the ground

Setup

Athletes stand on chairs or a park bench with a flat and clear landing area in front of them.

Execution

An athlete begins by repeatedly jumping off the chair or bench and landing in the open space in front of it. After several jumps, ask the athlete to begin to notice the landing position each time he or she jumps off the chair. Proper landing position should put athletes on the balls of their feet with knees slightly bent, buttocks in almost a sitting position, head up, and arms bent at 90-degree angles at the elbows. Athletes experience how their bodies feel when they execute a proper landing and become prepared to execute the progressions correctly. Three progressions advance from a simple jump off a chair with a controlled landing and positioning of the athlete's feet to more advanced turns and landing positions.

Progression 1

This progression trains the body to become aware and to maintain control in motion. Athletes jump from a chair or bench *(a)*. Using hips, arms, and shoulders to twist the body *(b)*, the athlete attempts to land with feet square and pointing 90 degrees to the left of the bench *(c)*. Repeat to the right side. Make note of where their feet are positioned at landing. The objective is to land consistently with feet squarely placed 90 degrees to the right or left of the bench.

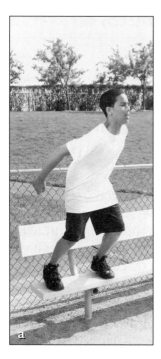 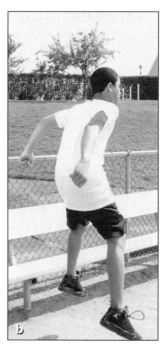 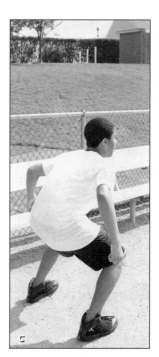

Progression 2

To emphasize body awareness, incorporate a challenge by requiring athletes to close their eyes during this progression. This forces the body to estimate and feel the correct adjustments that must be made rather than relying on sight. Jumping from a bench, the athlete closes the eyes and attempts to land with feet squarely pointing 90 degrees to the right of the bench. Repeat to the left.

Progression 3

This progression improves body awareness by increasing the difficulty of the jump. An athlete jumps off a bench *(a)*, turns 180 degrees in the air, and lands facing the bench *(b)*. Athletes attempt to land with both feet squarely facing the bench each time. Emphasize landing in the proper position.

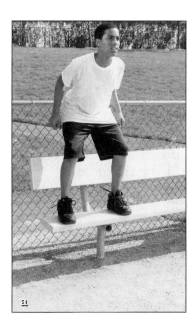 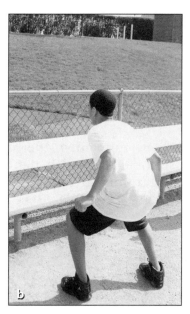

Three-Legged Moves

Age Range

8 to 14

Purpose

To improve on getting athletes into athletic positions; to help athletes move in the kind of unusual body positions they find themselves in during competition

Benefits

During sport, athletes are often placed in situations that can be uncomfortable or unfamiliar, and yet they must perform. Some athletes have a difficult time getting low and moving because they lack flexibility and overall body awareness. The more flexible the body is, the more effective maneuvers will be during competition. This drill is the first phase in training the body to get into an athletic position to execute standard moves.

Equipment

A 3-inch cone or rubber dot, an 8-inch cone, a 15-inch cone, a 2-foot cone

Setup

Mark a starting line three yards from the first cone and a finish line three yards from the last cone or dot. Set up the cones about three yards apart in a straight row. The cones must vary in size.

Execution

Each athlete runs down the line, places a hand on the first cone, and (with hand still on cone) runs 360 degrees around the cone before advancing to the next one. The athlete repeats the move until he or she finishes circling all four cones and crosses the finish line.

Competition

Record how long it takes athletes to complete the course. Add two seconds for every cone from which the hand slips off during the 360-degree spin. Athletes measure progress by establishing a personal-best time after completing five course runs. From then on, they receive 1 point for every quarter-second under their personal best.

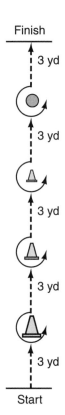

Finish

3 yd

3 yd

3 yd

3 yd

3 yd

3 yd

Start

Multiple and Continuous Movements

Age Range

8 to 14

Purpose

To develop a sense of how to move and to readjust movements under multiple competitive situations

Benefits

Most sports place athletes in situations in which they must execute multiple movements at once, or one right after another, during the flow of competition, so it's important that they practice executing multiple movements simultaneously. This drill helps athletes develop multiple-movement skills.

Equipment

Eight cones, three 6-inch minihurdles, a tumbling mat

Setup

Place one cone on the ground three feet in front of a tumbling mat. This will be the starting point. Place a cone five yards from the opposite side of the tumbling mat. On the starting-line side of the mat, place three six-inch hurdles about two feet apart and then a cone three feet from the last hurdle. Place another cone five yards away from the last cone as the finish line (see diagram).

Execution

This drill involves two progressions that emphasize multiple movements and continuous body readjustments.

Progression 1

Starting from a standing position and facing the mat, an athlete executes a forward roll onto the mat. The athlete then immediately steps off the mat and runs to a cone five yards away. He or she does a 360-degree turn with one hand placed on the cone. The athlete then returns to the mat on the opposite side of the starting line for a second forward roll. The athlete then steps off the mat and strides over three consecutive minihurdles about two feet apart. This is followed by a second 360-degree turn around the cone three feet from the last hurdle (hand remains on the cone during the turn). The athlete finishes by running past the finish line five yards past the cone. Emphasize a smooth transition between movements and keeping the body completely controlled.

Competition

Time how long it takes for athletes to complete the course. Add two seconds for each hurdle missed and also for each cone an athlete doesn't maintain

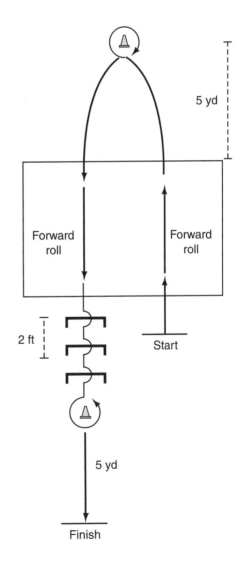

contact with during the 360-degree turns. Athletes execute the course five times, taking their best time as their base time. On subsequent runs, they receive 5 points for every half-second faster than their previous best.

Progression 2

Repeat progression 1 but add four cones placed in a zigzag arrangement (three yards apart) at the end of the course. End with each athlete touching each cone with one hand (without circling) down the course.

Competition

Time how long it takes for athletes to complete the course. Add two seconds for each hurdle missed, for each cone the athlete doesn't maintain contact with during the turns, and for every cone not touched to finish the course. Athletes execute the course five times, taking the best time as their base time. On subsequent runs, they receive 5 points for every half-second faster than their previous best.

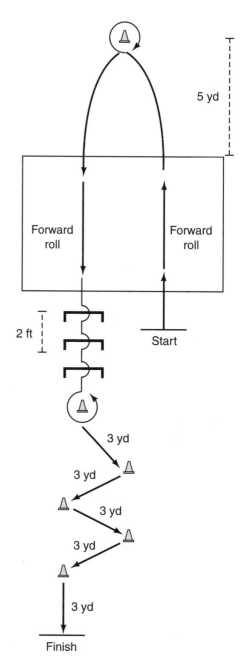

▬ Quick Feet ▬

Age Range

8 to 14

Purpose

To improve overall foot movement

Benefits

Every sport involves lower-body movement. Athletes who perfect their efficiency of movement to get to a particular spot on the field, court, or ice before an opponent and place themselves in a position to execute are those who experience more overall success.

Equipment

Agility ladder (or draw squares with chalk on pavement—eight consecutive squares about a foot wide and a foot long), four cones

Setup

Athletes begin at one end of the agility ladder and finish at the other end.

Execution

Three progressions advance the continuous movement of the feet. Note that we'll focus on a series of lower-body movements in most of our agility drills:

- Lateral movement—feet slide across but never cross each other, barely touching during each stride of a shuffle-type movement; arms stay close to the body and slightly bent at the elbows; hips and shoulders remain square, with weight distributed on the balls of the feet;
- Crossover movement—feet cross by alternating front and back in a quick motion; hips and shoulders remain square; weight is on the balls of the feet; arms are close to the body and slightly bent; arms do not swing across the body;
- Backpedaling—weight is on the balls of the feet; waist is bent slightly forward; arms swing back rapidly and close to the body. (See chapter 8 for proper backpedaling technique.)

Progression 1

Athletes start by running down one side of the ladder. They place two feet in each square of the ladder and then immediately move to the next square, progressing until they finish. Watch for kids looking at their feet while executing this drill. This is natural at first. After several repetitions, tell them to keep their heads up and eyes forward as they cross the ladder.

Competition

Time how long it takes for athletes to complete the course. Add one second for each failed attempt to place two feet in each box. Athletes execute the course five times, taking their best time as their base time. On subsequent runs, they receive 5 points for every half-second faster than their previous best.

Progression 2

This progression combines the quick forward movement of the lower body with quick lateral movements as athletes transition into different positions.

Each athlete starts by facing the eight-step ladder laid flat on the ground. The athlete takes two steps per ladder square for two consecutive squares, followed immediately by laterally moving to the outside of the ladder on the right and touching an eight-inch cone before moving laterally back into the ladder with two immediate steps. The athlete then continues to move forward up the ladder, taking two steps in the next square and again moving outside the ladder, this time to the left, and touching another eight-inch cone before repeating the sequences until finishing the ladder. Placing smaller cones on the outside of the ladder increases the difficulty.

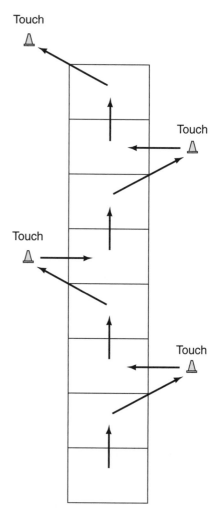

Competition

Time how long it takes for athletes to complete the course. Add one second for each failed attempt to place two feet in each box or for each missed execution of a lateral or forward move. Athletes execute the course five times, taking the best time as their base time. On subsequent runs, they receive 5 points for every half-second faster than their previous best.

Progression 3

In this progression we incorporate several quick movements (backpedal, lateral steps, forward steps) to help athletes develop a rhythm and feel for moving with different coordinated moves.

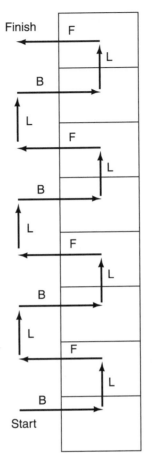

Each athlete starts with his or her back to the agility ladder. The athlete steps backward into the first box, quickly takes two steps in place, and then immediately moves laterally to the right (hips will be square to the left side of the ladder). After taking only two steps in place, the athlete then immediately moves forward out of the ladder. He or she takes two quick steps in place and moves laterally to the right, adjacent to the next square up the ladder with the athlete's back to the ladder and hips square. The athlete takes only two steps, followed by backpedaling into the ladder, and then repeats each sequence of movements until finishing all eight ladder squares.

Watch that athletes take only two steps in each square before moving to the next spot; this creates a rhythm that they can pick up on and perfect. Also be sure that they execute each move while keeping shoulders and hips square.

🎖 Competition

Time how long it takes athletes to complete the course. Add one second for each failed attempt to place two feet in each box or for improper execution of a backpedal, lateral, or forward move. Athletes execute the course five times, taking the best time as their base time. On subsequent runs, they receive 5 points for every half-second faster than their previous best.

Crossing the Feet

Age Range

8 to 14

Purpose

To improve footwork

Benefits

Most sports require parts of the lower body to quickly cross in order to start or change direction (think of an infielder's first step to field a ground ball, a hockey player suddenly changing direction, or a lacrosse player avoiding a defender). This drill exaggerates the movement with multiple switching of the feet both across the front and behind to familiarize the body to the movement.

Equipment

Eight cones

Setup

Arrange eight cones on the ground in two rows 5 yards across from each other. In the left row, three cones are placed 10 yards apart; in the right row, five cones are placed 5 yards apart (see diagram on page 156).

Execution

Two progressions work on lateral movement and crossing the feet while moving laterally in both directions.

Progression 1

Athletes begin by moving from cone A to cone B by quickly crossing the left foot across the right foot *(a)*. This is followed by the right foot sliding back parallel to the left foot so that the legs are no longer crossed *(b)*. Athletes then immediately cross the left foot behind the right foot, followed by the right foot sliding back parallel to the left foot. They continue until reaching cone B and then return to cone A by repeating movement in the opposite direction.

Progression 2

Athletes build on the first part of the drill after mastering the basic movement in both directions. Athletes start at cone A and cross feet left to right to cone B. They then return in the opposite direction from cone B to cone A, pivot, and cross feet left to right at an angle to cone C, pivot again, and cross feet at an angle right to left to cone

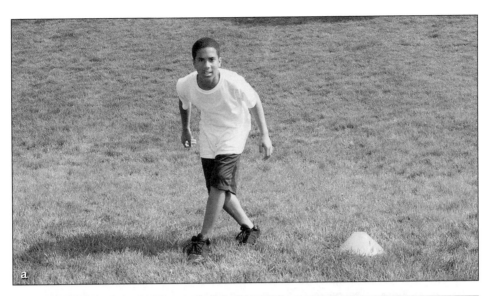

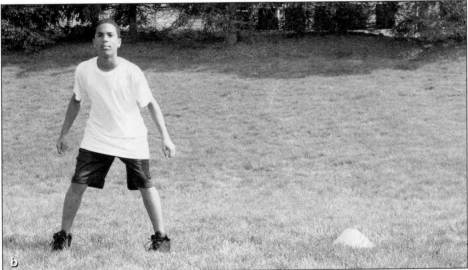

D. They then cross feet left to right to cone E and return by crossing feet in the opposite direction back to cone D, pivot, and cross feet left to right at an angle to cone F. They then pivot and cross feet at an angle right to left to cone G, cross feet left to right to cone H, and return in the opposite direction from cone H to finish at cone G.

Competition

Time how long it takes for athletes to complete the course. Athletes execute the course five times, taking the best time as their base time. In subsequent passes through the course, they receive 5 points for every half-second faster than their previous best time.

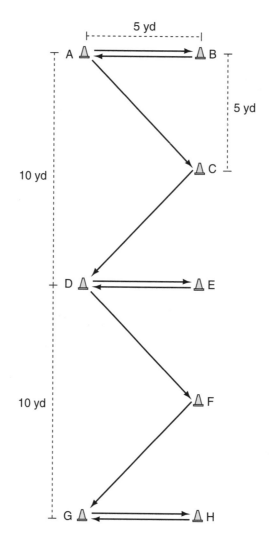

DRILL 9.6
30-Yard Athletic Slalom

Age Range

8 to 14

Purpose

To improve agility of movement by duplicating sport-specific movements upfield

Benefits

This drill benefits movement in field sports such as football, lacrosse, and soccer. Very rarely in field sports does an athlete run straight downfield. More often, the pattern of running tests the agility of the athlete repeatedly and throughout the course of competition. This drill attempts to duplicate agility moves an athlete might face when maneuvering up a field of play.

Equipment

Four orange cones, three blue cones

Setup

Mark a start line and place an orange cone (cone A) five yards directly upfield. Place a blue cone (cone B) two yards to the right. Place an orange cone (cone C) three yards to the left of cone B. Place an orange cone (cone D) five yards directly upfield from cone C. Place a blue cone (cone E) two yards to the right of cone D. Place an orange cone (cone F) three yards to the left of cone E. Place a final blue cone (cone G) five yards upfield and two yards to the right of cone F. Mark a finish line five yards upfield from cone G.

Execution

Athletes complete the drill as quickly as possible by successfully maneuvering through the course. They must go left around all orange cones and right around all blue cones. They begin by running around the left side of cone A and immediately to cone B. They circle around the right of cone B and proceed around the left of cone C. They then go directly upfield around the left of cone D and progress to the right around the right side of cone E. They then run left around the left side of cone F and then right around the right side of cone G before finishing directly upfield from cone G at the finish line. We recommend running the competition in the opposite direction to duplicate movements downfield.

Specific sport elements such as carrying a football and switching to the correct hand, handling a lacrosse sick and cradling a ball, or dribbling a soccer ball through the course can be included to increase the difficulty of the drill.

🎗 Competition

Time how long it takes to run the course, adding two seconds for every cone missed and another two seconds for cones run in the wrong direction.

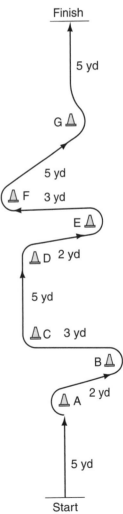

Stop, Cut, and Go

Age Range

8 to 14

Purpose

To improve total body control

Benefits

In football, lacrosse, and soccer, an effective move when confronting a defender on the field is a spin or 180-degree turn followed immediately by moving away from the opponent. This move requires athletes to quickly stop their forward motion, plant their pivot foot, and spin until they're open to move to open space. This drill simulates an important move that should be in every athlete's repertoire.

Equipment

Seven cones

Setup

Cone A serves as a starting line. Place cone B 10 yards from the starting line and cone C 5 yards upfield from cone B. Place cone D 5 yards to the left of cone C and another 5 yards upfield. Place cone E 5 yards to the right of cone D and another 5 yards upfield. Finally, place a finish line marked by two cones 5 yards upfield from cone E.

Execution

Each athlete starts at the starting line at cone A and runs 10 yards upfield to cone B. The athlete plants the left foot in front of cone B (which is simulating an opponent) and pivots with a spin that positions the back to the cone and moves the body around the left side of the cone. The athlete then immediately sprints to the front of cone C, where he or she plants the right foot in front of the cone and pivots with the back facing the cone, moving to the right side of the cone until reaching the opposite side of the cone. The athlete then sprints to cone D, plants the left

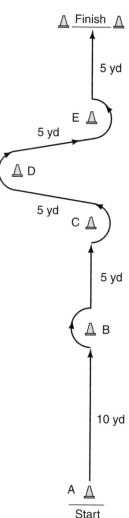

foot, and pivots with the back to the cone around the left side of the cone. The athlete sprints to cone E, where he or she plants the right foot, pivots, and spins with the back to the cone and moves around to the right of the cone before sprinting to the finish.

🎗 Competition

To execute the competition for football and lacrosse, be sure to hold the ball and stick in the correct hand when turning and running upfield. Scores are determined by timing the course using the correct plant foot and turn. Add three seconds to the final time for each incorrect plant and turn.

Run & Shoot and Run & Throw

Age Range

8 to 14

Purpose

To improve execution of baseball, football, and lacrosse skills while in motion

Benefits

This drill emphasizes quick footwork in combination with stabilizing and controlling the body to execute sport-specific skills

Equipment

Six cones; lacrosse goal or a baseball diamond backstop (with a three-foot by three-foot square marked by tape); one rubber dot for soccer; five baseballs; five footballs; five lacrosse balls; five soccer balls; a lacrosse stick

Setup

Place three cones in a horizontal row five yards apart (cones F, A, and B). Place another cone (cone D) five yards in front of cone A. Place another cone (cone C) at a 45-degree angle five yards away from cone A. Place a final cone (cone E) at a 135-degree angle from

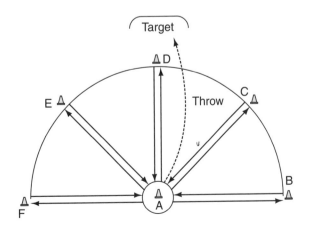

cone A. Position cone D five yards from a baseball backstop or a fence for baseball, football, or soccer skills, and a lacrosse goal five yards behind cone D for lacrosse skills.

Baseball or Football

An athlete starts at cone A and then runs and picks up a baseball or football at cone B (note that the athlete's body should not be facing the target behind cone D). The athlete returns to cone A and throws to hit the target behind cone D. Be sure athletes makes their throws at cone A, not prior to reaching the cone. Athletes continue to execute the same movement and throws continuously from cone C to cone F. Emphasize to athletes that they should make their throws without hesitating as soon as they reach cone A.

Competition

Time how long it takes athletes to complete the course. Subtract two seconds for every target they hit.

Soccer

Duplicate the execution for baseball and football but dribble a soccer ball back to a flat rubber dot at point A each time before kicking the ball toward the target.

Competition

Time how long it takes athletes to complete the course. Subtract two seconds for every target they hit.

Lacrosse

Duplicate the execution for baseball and football but change the target to a lacrosse goal.

Competition

Time how long it takes athletes to complete the course. Subtract two seconds for every target they hit.

Sport-
Specific
Drill

DRILL 9.9
Soccer Agility

Age Range

8 to 14

Purpose

To increase overall agility in combination with ball control and footwork

Benefits

Athletes develop footwork and lower-body control.

Equipment

Five soccer balls, 25 cones

Setup

Arrange five soccer balls two yards apart in a straight horizontal row. Upfield from each ball (five total rows) there is a vertical row of five cones placed a yard apart (see diagram).

Execution

An athlete starts by tapping the top of soccer ball A with each foot before traveling down the line and tapping the top of each ball with each foot, keeping each ball stationary until reaching the last ball (ball E). After tapping ball E twice, the athlete dribbles around the five cones placed one yard apart in front of ball E, leaves the ball at the end of the row of cones, and continues running around all cones to the right until reaching ball A again. The athlete repeats, tapping each ball twice on top from ball A to ball D, keeping each ball stationary until reaching the last ball on the row (ball D). The athlete taps twice

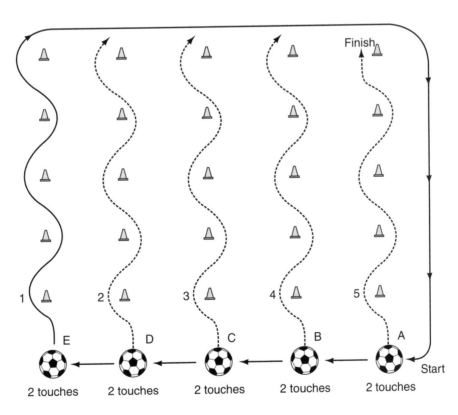

on top of ball D and then dribbles through the five cones in front of ball D. This rotation continues until the final ball (ball A) is tapped twice and dribbled through the final five cones.

Competition

Time how long it takes athletes to complete the course; add one second for each ball not tapped twice and each cone missed or knocked over.

Appendix A
Metric Conversions

The drills in this book use English measurements. To convert measurements to metric, refer to the following lists. Conversions are given for the measurements of distance and weight used in the drills. Note that conversion measurements are rounded to the nearest tenth.

Distance

Inches (in.) to Centimeters (cm)

1 in. = 2.5 cm
2 in. = 5.1 cm
3 in. = 7.6 cm
4 in. = 10.2 cm
5 in. = 12.7 cm
6 in. = 15.2 cm
7 in. = 17.8 cm
8 in. = 20.3 cm
9 in. = 22.9 cm
10 in. = 25.4 cm
15 in. = 38.1 cm
20 in. = 50.8 cm
25 in. = 63.5 cm

Feet (ft) to Meters (m)

1 ft = 0.3 m
2 ft = 0.6 m
3 ft = 0.9 m
4 ft = 1.2 m
5 ft = 1.5 m
6 ft = 1.8 m
7 ft = 2.1 m
8 ft = 2.4 m
9 ft = 2.7 m

10 ft = 3 m
25 ft = 7.6 m
50 ft = 15.2 m

Yards (yd) to Meters (m)

1 yd = 0.9 m
2 yd = 1.8 m
3 yd = 2.7 m
4 yd = 3.7 m
5 yd = 4.6 m
6 yd = 5.5 m
7 yd = 6.4 m
8 yd = 7.3 m
9 yd = 8.2 m
10 yd = 9.1 m
25 yd = 22.9 m
50 yd = 45.7 m

Weight

Pounds (lb) to Kilograms (kg)

1 lb = 0.5 kg
2 lb = 0.9 kg
3 lb = 1.4 kg
4 lb = 1.8 kg
5 lb = 2.3 kg
6 lb = 2.7 kg
7 lb = 3.2 kg
8 lb = 3.6 kg
9 lb = 4.1 kg
10 lb = 4.5 kg
11 lb = 5.0 kg
12 lb = 5.4 kg
13 lb = 5.9 kg
14 lb = 6.4 kg
15 lb = 6.8 kg

Appendix B
Throwing Tips

Although they are not comprehensive, the following tips help young athletes accurately and effectively execute the throwing skills employed in the drills and competitions. It's important that athletes use efficient throwing form when executing the drills so that they build muscle memory and develop proper throwing habits.

How to Throw a Baseball

To throw a baseball with accuracy and consistency, an athlete must point the nonthrowing shoulder at the target. Be sure athletes keep their shoulders horizontal to the ground to ensure accuracy. The throwing arm must keep the elbow above the shoulder. Although athletes tend to vary in their delivery, it's usually best to throw a ball from over the top rather than sidearm. The over-the-top and the three-quarter arm movement are the two most common and recommended techniques for accuracy and consistency. When the ball is released from the hand, the front foot (left foot for right-handers) should be planted on the ground with the back foot pushing off on the ball of the foot.

For a short accurate throw (such as from shortstop to first base), an athlete should get as much momentum moving toward the target as possible. This is accomplished by shuffling the feet toward the target (the feet should not cross, nor should the athlete hop to keep the shoulders horizontal), cutting down the distance between the athlete and the target. After the shuffle toward the target and throw, the athlete continues to move toward the intended target by following the throw; this emphasizes the forward throwing motion.

For longer throws (such as from left field to home), athletes should use the entire body to create as much power as possible. This is accomplished by creating momentum when preparing to throw by taking several strong steps followed by a slight hop and a step-through toward the target. The step-through involves the proper transfer of weight from the back foot (right foot for right-handers) to the front foot with a strong over-the-top throw.

How to Throw a Football

There is one standard way to throw a football. An athlete holds the ball with fingers spread over the laces and the index finger extended toward the tip of the ball. Proper throwing position begins with the feet shoulder-width apart and the nonthrowing shoulder pointed at the target.

The ball is brought back into the throwing position with two hands by pushing the ball directly back to the ear, with the back of the ball pointing in a straight line directly behind the thrower. Before the throw, the athlete's weight should be slightly shifted onto the back foot. When the throw begins, the lower body moves first, transferring weight from the back foot onto the front foot, with hips and shoulders following and squaring up with the front foot. The athlete's weight then rolls onto the front of the front foot. His or her nonthrowing arm comes off the football and continues around the body, pulling the throwing arm through. The throwing arm follows the ball as it leaves the hand with the index finger pointing toward the target and palm facing the ground.

How to Throw a Lacrosse Ball

Throwing a lacrosse ball is similar to throwing a baseball. An athlete should hold the stick with the head positioned to the ear of the throwing side. Shoulders should stay perpendicular to the target as the athlete points the off-stick shoulder at the target. Begin the throw by positioning the top hand near the head of the stick; throw with the top hand, pull with the bottom hand, and step with the front foot toward the target. The athlete follows through with the stick finishing with the head pointing toward the target and the stick parallel to the ground. The top hand is usually the athlete's dominant throwing hand.

About the Authors

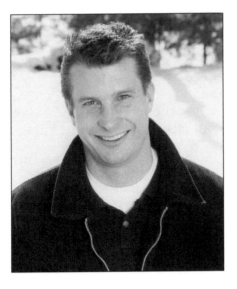

Scott Lancaster is the founder and CEO of Youth Evolution Sports (www.youthevolutionsports.com), a multimedia, content, and youth sports marketing company that services kids, parents, coaches, corporations, and major league sport organizations. He has developed youth sport programs for the past 19 years, both in affiliation with U.S. Soccer and as the former senior director of youth football for the National Football League. The author of *Fair Play*, he has been interviewed by numerous media outlets, including the NBC *Today Show*, CNN, the CBS *Early Show*, the *New York Times*, the *Chicago Tribune*, the *Boston Globe*, National Public Radio, *Woman's Day*, and *Ladies' Home Journal*. He also hosts his own national youth sports radio show, *The ABCs of Sports*, for parents and coaches on Sirius Radio, channel 123.

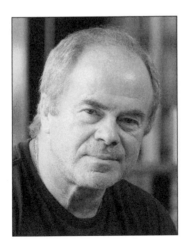

Radu Teodorescu runs a training center in New York City, where he has trained everyone from children to celebrities, including Jennifer Lopez, Candice Bergen, Matthew Broderick, and Vanessa Williams. Teodorescu has been featured in more than 400 magazine articles and has spoken at conferences and given fitness clinics across the United States. He is widely known for creating, writing, and producing videos with celebrity model and fitness enthusiast Cindy Crawford, including *Shape Your Body*, which is the best-selling fitness video of all time.

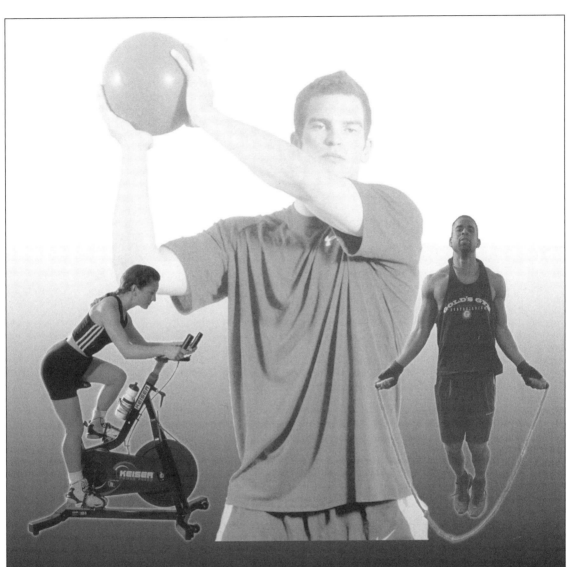